Dad Rookie

The Game-Changing Pregnancy Guide for
First-Time Dads

Lane Carter

For Claire, Jack, and Lane................

You are my greatest adventure, my proudest achievement, and my deepest joy. Thank you for filling my life with laughter, love, and purpose. You inspire me everyday, and I'm forever grateful and blessed to be your dad.

Contents

Introduction

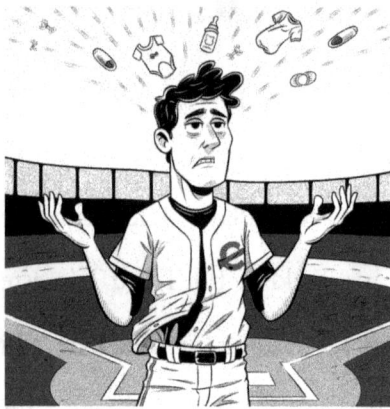

I remember standing in the baby store, surrounded by cribs, strollers, and tiny socks, feeling like I'd just been thrown into a championship game without knowing the rules. The sales associate was chatting away about swaddling techniques and diaper brands, but all I could think about was how I'd never even held a baby before. The realization hit me like I was standing flat-footed in left field, the fly ball heading my way, and I had no clue what to do with the ball or what the score was.

I was about to become a father, and I had no idea what I was doing!

If you're reading this, you might be in a similar spot. Maybe you're expecting your first child, or perhaps you're holding a positive pregnancy test in your hand, feeling thrilled and terrified at the same time. My goal with this book is to help you take on the challenge with confidence and a bit of humor. *Dad Rookie: The Game-Changing Pregnancy Guide for First-Time Dads* is your ultimate playbook, designed to coach you through the playoffs of parenthood and get you game-ready for the big moments ahead.

This book's purpose is straightforward: to be an easy-to-read, informative guide for first-time dads. I want to arm you with practical knowledge and insights so you can face fatherhood with assurance. You'll find tips from dealing with morning sickness (not yours, hopefully) to changing diapers like a pro. Each chapter is designed to boost your confidence and equip you with the resources you need to be an engaged, supportive dad.

Why am I so passionate about this? Because I know firsthand the challenges and joys of early fatherhood. I've seen too many new dads feel overwhelmed and underprepared, and I want to change that. I want to empower you with the confidence and skills that will make your rookie season of fatherhood not just survivable but truly enjoyable. Being a dad is one of the most important positions you'll ever take, and I'm here to help you nail it.

Throughout the book, you'll find insights into the three stages of pregnancy, how to support your wife or partner during each trimester, and what to expect when the baby arrives. We'll cover newborn care with step-by-step instructions for tasks like bathing, swaddling, and feeding. You'll learn techniques for bonding and connecting with your baby and strategies for maintaining an intimate relationship with your partner. Emotional health and stress management are also key focuses, as is understanding modern parenting roles and shared responsibilities.

This book is for men expecting their first child or new to fatherhood. You're in the right place if you're looking for guidance on pregnancy, newborn care, and effective parenting. Whether you're a nervous first-time dad or just looking to improve your parenting skills, this guide has the perfect plays and strategies for you.

What sets this book apart? It doesn't just cover baby basics. It also deals with understanding the modern role of dads in today's diverse family structures. You'll find expert insights, stories from dads who've been there, and practical advice tailored to contemporary parenting. The checklists and summaries in each chapter are designed to help you apply what you learn, making the information as actionable as possible.

I encourage you to engage with this book actively. Use the checklists, jot down notes, and share your favorite pro tips with fellow dads-to-be. Think of fatherhood as your championship run—it's the biggest, most rewarding challenge you'll ever tackle. Much like a rookie athlete stepping onto the field for the first time, as a new dad, you'll be building new skills, learning the playbook day by day, and stepping up to a major league responsibility. Embrace it with excitement and enthusiasm. You've got this!

Fatherhood is a game filled with unknowns, tough calls, and unexpected plays, but also packed with victories and unforgettable moments. This playbook is here to break down your everyday questions, giving you the game plan and tools you need to handle pregnancy and early parenthood like a pro. So, let's hit the ground running. Together, we'll turn those rookie jitters into confidence, gearing you up for the ultimate season—fatherhood.

Bonus Gift

Before we officially kick off your *Dad Rookie* training, I want to give you something.

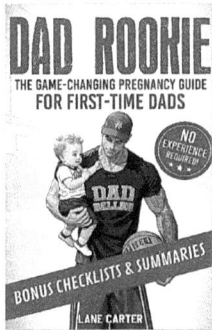

As you step onto the field of fatherhood, I know there are a lot of plays to learn and challenges ahead. From supporting your wife or partner during pregnancy, to bonding with your little teammate, mastering new dad skills, packing the right gear for the hospital, and planning for new family expenses—it's a whole new ballgame.

That's why I've put together a complimentary handbook—a quick-reference, go-to guide packed with the checklists and step-by-step strategies provided throughout this book to help you navigate pregnancy and the first six months with your baby. This is the reference guide I wish I had during my own rookie season as a dad.

It's filled with the following pro tips and must-know moves to keep you in control of the game:

- Third Trimester Health Checklist

- Birth Plan Worksheet

- Ultimate Mom/Baby Hospital Bag Checklist

- Newborn Sleep, Feeding, & Wake Patterns

- Diaper Duty Step-by-Step Guide

- Baby Changing Station Checklist

- How to Swaddle a Baby Guide

- Paternal Postpartum Depression Symptoms List

- New Family Expenses List

Best part? You can download it for <u>free</u> and have it ready in your dad gear bag whenever you need it.

Utilizing the camera on your mobile device, just scan the QR code above and click the link that pops up. It will take you directly to the Dad Rookie Bonus Checklists & Summaries.

Now, let's get the training started and you game-ready!

1

Game On – Breaking Down Pregnancy and the First Trimester

The day my wife told me she was pregnant, I was kicked back on our beat-up couch, mindlessly flipping through channels like it was halftime. She casually handed me a small, white stick with two pink lines on it. At first, I thought it was some kind of new fitness tracker.

Then it hit me.

My heart started pounding like I was stepping up to the plate in the bottom of the ninth with two outs. This was it—the start of the biggest season of my life.

If you're anything like me, the first trimester is when the game plan starts forming, and the questions start piling up. *What's actually happening inside that incredible belly? How do I step up and be the best teammate possible for my wife through all these changes?*

This chapter is your pregame warm-up, breaking down the first three months of pregnancy and the fast-paced action that comes with it.

First trimester overview: What to expect

The first trimester—first three months, aka the first quarter in guy terms—is like the opening drive of a game, setting the stage for everything that follows. It's a time of immense change for your partner and you. Her body is working overtime, and her hormones are having a party—bringing along guests like nausea, fatigue, and mood swings. These hormones, while vital for fetal development, can turn life into a bit of a rollercoaster. You might notice her craving pickles and ice cream one day and feeling too queasy to eat the next. It's all part of the process. Early prenatal care is important during this time as it provides a chance to monitor the baby's development and address any health concerns that may arise. Regular check-ups ensure that both Mom and Baby are thriving, providing peace of mind for everyone involved.

Emotionally, for the both of you, expect a mixed bag of excitement, fear, and everything in between. You might feel anxious about the changes ahead, and that's perfectly normal. She will likely experience a range of emotions as her body and mind adjust to the pregnancy. It's important to handle these feelings together, approaching them with empathy and understanding. Moods might swing like a pendulum, and early pregnancy anxieties may crop up unexpectedly. Your role here isn't to have all the answers but to be a steady presence, offering reassurance and a listening ear when needed.

Your wife or partner will appreciate the support, both emotional and physical, as she experiences these changes. Whether offering to handle more household chores or simply being there to discuss her concerns, your involvement makes a difference. Active participation in prenatal activities sets the tone for a supportive partnership. Attending prenatal appointments will allow you to hear the baby's heartbeat for the first time—a moment that can solidify the reality of what's happening. Engaging in pregnancy-related reading (like this book!) will give you a better understanding of what she's experiencing, making conversations more meaningful. Don't underestimate the power of helping with baby prep; picking out tiny clothes and assembling a crib can be surprisingly bonding experiences and a tangible way to contribute.

Fetal development in the first trimester: Month-by-month guide

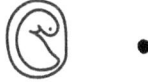

The first trimester is a period of extraordinary transformation for your little one. At the beginning of the very first month, the baby is no bigger than a grain of sand. By month end, they're still smaller than a piece of rice yet monumental changes are taking place within this tiny speck. It all starts with the formation of the major organs. By the end of the first month, the heart begins to beat, and the foundation for the fetus' brain and spinal cord is being laid. You might think of it as the blueprint phase of construction, where everything essential is planned out. This is also when those limb buds appear, which will eventually grow into arms and legs—a reminder that a whole person is developing inside that growing belly.

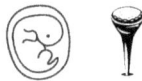

At the beginning of the second month, the embryo is about the size of a golf tee head. Facial features start to form, with the beginnings of eyes, nostrils, and ears first appearing. The brain continues to develop rapidly, and you might even catch a glimpse of these changes during an ultrasound. It's incredible to think that so much is happening at such a microscopic level, yet these developments are essential for the baby's health and well-being. As these features take shape, your partner might notice her emotions fluctuating more as her body adapts to these changes.

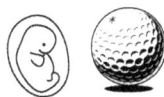

By the end of the third month, the transition from embryo to fetus is complete. The fetus is slightly larger than a golf ball, and small movements begin, although your wife or partner won't feel them just yet. This is also when reflexes start to develop. Imagine your little one moving their tiny fingers or toes for the first time. These movements are a rehearsal for life outside the womb, preparing the baby for the world ahead. Meanwhile, your partner may continue to experience the physical demands of nurturing this rapidly growing life, sometimes feeling fatigued or queasy.

Understanding these milestones can help you connect with your partner's experience. Each development inside the womb can mirror the changes she feels on the outside. It's like impressive gameplay coming together perfectly. You might want to use interactive pregnancy apps to track fetal development to support this understanding. They are an excellent resource for providing weekly updates on the baby's size and growth. They also offer fascinating insights to help you visualize the baby's progress. These tools keep you informed plus they can enhance your bond with your baby. As you learn more about what's happening inside the womb, you'll find it easier to engage with your partner and share in the excitement of each new milestone.

Pregnancy playbook: Spotting common symptoms and supporting like a pro

Pregnancy can feel like a whirlwind, and the first trimester often brings a host of symptoms that can catch both of you off guard. Morning sickness is likely the first hurdle you'll encounter, and despite its name, it can strike at any hour. To help alleviate this, keep ginger ale or crackers handy; they can be lifesavers when nausea hits. Fatigue might also become a constant companion during this time. Don't be surprised if she suddenly falls asleep on the couch during a movie you both were excited to watch. You'll also notice changes in her eating patterns, from aversions to foods she once loved to unexpected cravings. It's all part of the body's way of adjusting, so be patient and ready to make a late-night run for Chinese takeout or watermelon if necessary.

Empathy and patience are your best allies during these first few months. You might not be able to physically feel what she's going through but understanding and patience can make all the difference. She is dealing with a complex blend of emotions and physical changes, so being there to listen and support is invaluable. You might notice she's more irritable or emotional than usual, which can be challenging. Remember, it's not personal; it's the hormones talking. Approach these moments with a calm demeanor and a willingness to help.

Strengthening the team bond in the first quarter

Building a strong connection with your wife or partner during pregnancy is like laying the foundation for a house. It's crucial for supporting the structure that will hold you both through the ups and downs of parenthood. This connection doesn't just benefit the two of you; it also creates a nurturing environment for your developing baby. When she feels supported and understood, it can positively impact her well-being and the baby's development. One of the best ways to strengthen this bond is through shared activities that promote relaxation and togetherness. What about setting aside time for date nights focused on unwinding? It doesn't have to be anything extravagant. A simple evening walk or cooking dinner together can work wonders. Participating in prenatal yoga classes is another fantastic way to connect. Yoga promotes physical health and also offers a shared experience that reinforces your partnership. These moments allow you to communicate on a deeper level, discussing your hopes and fears about parenthood in a relaxed setting.

Productive communication is the glue that holds this emotional connection together. It's important to maintain an open and honest dialogue throughout the pregnancy. This means creating a safe space for you both to express your feelings without judgment. One approach is to set aside regular times to talk about any concerns you might have. This will help prevent misunderstandings and ensure you're both on the same page. Sometimes, knowing that she is there to listen—and really hears you—can be incredibly reassuring.

Pregnancy can also present emotional challenges that require attention and care. Stress and anxiety might rear their heads, and it's essential to recognize and address them early. As a dad-to-be, offering reassurance and support can make a significant difference. Remind her that it's okay to feel overwhelmed or afraid and that you're in this together. Sometimes, the simple act of being present and attentive is all it takes to lighten the emotional load. If stress becomes too much, consider exploring stress management techniques together. Practicing mindfulness or engaging in light physical activities can alleviate some tension. Remember, the goal is not to fix everything but to be a constant and comforting presence in your partner's life.

Running a solid game plan: Effective communication during pregnancy

Communication is the lifeline of any relationship, but it takes on an even more significant role during pregnancy. It's the playbook that guides you both as you tackle this transformative time together. Effective communication keeps your partnership in sync, allowing you to express your needs, desires, and concerns openly. It helps you understand each other's perspectives and work through challenges as a team. Without it, misunderstandings can create penalties, leading to unnecessary stress.

To improve communication, try incorporating some practical skills into your daily interactions. Active listening is a great place to start. It involves more than just hearing words; it's about truly understanding what she is saying. Another technique is using "I" statements to express feelings.

Instead of saying, "You never listen to me," try, "I feel unheard when I'm talking." This approach focuses on your emotions without placing blame, generating a more empathetic dialogue.

Empathy is the cornerstone of meaningful conversations. It requires stepping into her shoes and acknowledging her feelings, even if you can't fully understand them. During pregnancy, she might be experiencing a whirlwind of emotions—joy, fear, excitement, and anxiety. Empathy involves recognizing these emotions and offering support without judgment. It means being there, not necessarily to solve every problem, but to listen and validate her experiences. This empathetic approach can transform your conversations into opportunities for connection rather than conflict.

As mentioned earlier, regular check-ins are also great for maintaining effective communication. Set aside time to discuss pregnancy and parenting expectations, perhaps during a quiet evening at home or a leisurely walk. Encourage each other to share your aspirations for the future and any anxieties that might be lurking in the background. These conversations provide a space for both of you to share your thoughts and feelings without distractions. They can help align your expectations and address concerns before they become major issues. Whether discussing your upcoming roles as parents or planning for the baby's arrival, regular check-ins keep you both on the same page, reinforcing your partnership.

Setting up the home field advantage (Creating a supportive home environment)

Visualize stepping into a place that immediately relaxes your mind and gets you in the zone—a place where stress seems to melt away, leaving only tranquility and comfort. This is the kind of home environment we want to create for you and your partner during pregnancy.

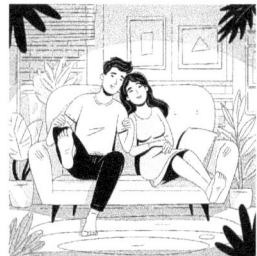

Practically, how can that be done? Start by decluttering and organizing your living space. A tidy home promotes a sense of calm, making everyday tasks feel less overwhelming. Organize items so everything has a place, reducing the chaos. If this task seems overwhelming, start room by room.

Shared responsibilities in the home are a game-changer. Pregnancy can be physically demanding, and sharing the load can alleviate some of the pressure on your mom-to-be. There are lots of tangible ways to lend a hand. Cooking simple but nutritious meals rich in essential nutrients can be a great start. Nutrition plays a major role in this stage. Foods high in calcium (think cheese and yogurt), protein (fish, poultry, meat, lentils, and beans), and iron (red meat, leafy greens, and dried fruit like prunes and raisins) are particularly important as they contribute to the baby's bone development and overall health.

Focus on making balanced dishes with plenty of fresh fruits, vegetables, and lean proteins, which can help sustain her energy and minimize nausea. If you're not much of a cook, try grilling a couple of pieces of chicken and serving them with a few boiled baby potatoes and a simple fresh salad. Or how about grabbing a packet of frozen stir-fry vegetables and some beef strips, stir fry them together in a wok and add some sweet and sour sauce? Game on! *Pro tip: a touch of ginger in the sauce will help quell her nausea.* Try making small, consistent choices that will contribute to your partner's health. Swap out the chips with the movie for air-popped popcorn or a bowl of unsalted nuts. Instead of bringing home a slab of chocolate, buy some dried fruit or jerky—great if she's nauseous.

Household chores are another area where you can step up. Whether taking over the vacuuming or keeping the kitchen tidy after dinner, these small acts of service can significantly lighten her load. Divide household duties in a way that feels fair and balanced to you both. You could take over the laundry or handle the grocery shopping. It's not just about getting things done; it's about sending a message that you're in this together and have her back. This cooperation can strengthen your bond and create a sense of teamwork that will serve you well into parenthood. Working together, even if you're just unloading the dishwasher and she's folding laundry, can be a rewarding experience, bringing you closer and making the challenges of pregnancy a little less daunting.

A healthy lifestyle extends beyond the physical. It's important to cultivate a positive atmosphere at home where she feels valued and cared for. Surprising her with her favorite snack or drawing a warm bath are little acts of kindness that can make a big difference. These gestures show her you're attentive to her needs and committed to making this time enjoyable and special. Remember, the environment you create now sets the tone for the months to come, laying the groundwork for a nurturing home where your family can thrive.

First quarter highlights: Key milestones of the first trimester

As we wrap up the first trimester, it's incredible to reflect on how much has happened in such a short period! Imagine a baseball, with a diameter of about 7.5 centimeters—this is the size of your growing baby by the end of these initial three months. What started as a single cell has blossomed into a complex little being. During this period, known as organogenesis, all the major organ systems have taken shape, setting the foundation for what will continue to develop in the months ahead. It's like watching a star athlete set up the perfect play, where every move builds toward a game-winning moment.

Your partner's connection with the baby grows stronger with each passing day. You'll witness a flickering heartbeat as you attend ultrasounds and perhaps even see tiny limbs in motion. These moments offer a tangible way to bond with your baby and transform abstract concepts into reality. Speak to the baby often; while they won't understand words yet, they will soon recognize familiar sounds at about 18 weeks. It's a simple yet profound way to begin forming a connection. This is when the magic of parenthood starts to feel real, as you begin to perceive the baby as a part of your family.

These early days also lay the groundwork for your relationship as co-parents. By actively participating in your wife's pregnancy, you're supporting her and building a team. These shared experiences will form the backbone of your parenting style, helping you handle future challenges with a united front. The small steps you take now, like attending medical appointments or reading about fetal development, are investments in your growing family. They enrich your understanding of what she is experiencing, show her that you're on board, and prepare you both for the exciting and sometimes unpredictable road ahead.

As you step into this new role, remember that each milestone is an opportunity to learn and grow. The first trimester is just the beginning—a time of rapid development and change for both the baby, your mom-to-be, and you. Embrace each moment with curiosity and openness, knowing you're laying a strong foundation for the months and years to come. This is a time of transformation—biologically, emotionally, and relationally. As you look forward to the following stages, carry with you the lessons and connections you've built, ready to face whatever comes your way with confidence and love.

2

Getting Ready for the Next Play – The Second Trimester

Second trimester: What to expect

The second trimester often sneaks up on you, like an opponent who can't miss a shot. One morning, you might find she has a bit more pep in her step, and you both realize some of the toughest parts of early pregnancy are behind you. It's great waking up to find that the constant nausea and fatigue have been replaced by a newfound surge of energy. It's like halftime, allowing you to catch your breath after the fast-paced first half. This is when you might notice your wife's glow—yes, it's real—and she might feel more like herself again. This phase, stretching from week 13 to week 26, is often considered the "honeymoon" period of pregnancy. It's a time when many women feel and look their best, and it's a great opportunity for you both to relish in the excitement of what's to come.

Morning sickness usually takes a seat on the bench as her energy levels rise. This shift means she might be more inclined to take on activities she enjoyed before pregnancy, from leisurely walks to light exercise. Encouraging her to engage in mild physical activities can help tackle common aches like back pain. You might incorporate short, daily walks into your routine. How about walking around the neighborhood together after dinner? Activities like this support physical health and offer a chance to connect and share in the pregnancy experience. As her body changes, sleep might still pose a challenge. Helping her find comfortable sleeping positions, like using a pregnancy pillow for support, can significantly affect her rest quality.

The second trimester is an ideal time to make the most of the energy and positivity you're both experiencing. Consider planning a "babymoon"—a final getaway before the baby arrives. It doesn't have to be extravagant; even a weekend road trip can offer the relaxation and bonding you need. This period is also perfect for capturing memories. Scheduling a maternity photoshoot can be a modern, fun, and meaningful way to document this special time. Many couples do this today and share this special time on social media. These photos will serve as reminders of the anticipation and joy you both felt as you prepared to welcome your little one.

Trimester progress: Breakdown of the baby's growth

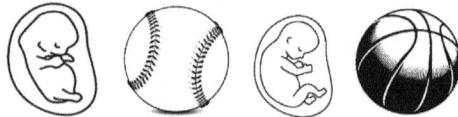

In the second trimester, it's as if the game picks up momentum—you can start to feel the action and see the plays come together. The fetus is baseball-sized at the start of the second trimester but transforms into something way more substantial by week 26. By the end of this trimester, your little one will be about the size of a standard basketball, and with each passing week, new milestones will unfold.

During this trimester, your baby is going through some incredible trans-formations. This is when they start to develop a more defined structure, with bones hardening and muscles strengthening. Around week 14, your baby's sex becomes apparent, a detail that adds a layer of excitement to the journey. By weeks 18 to 20, she might feel those first tiny flutters, known as quickening. These tiny movements are the baby's way of practicing coordination as they explore the expanding world around them. It's a time of active fetal growth, and you should see this progress during an ultrasound. These milestones are exciting and reassuring, as they signify healthy development.

As the weeks pass, your baby's senses begin to take shape. The eyes are developing, and by week 26, they might even start opening. Meanwhile, the ears are honing their ability to hear, meaning your voice can be a familiar comfort even before birth. Try talking or singing to the baby; it's a simple way to build a connection. If you play a musical instrument, you may want to play softly for your little one.

The once-soft skeleton continues to harden, and the skin begins to accumulate a fatty layer under it to provide insulation for the journey ahead. This is also when vernix, a white, waxy coating, and lanugo (fine hair) cover the fetus to protect its skin. These developments are vital as they aid in regulating body temperature and preparing the baby for life outside the womb.

Your partner's body will mirror these changes, adapting to support the baby's growth. As the baby becomes more active, you might notice her belly moving with little kicks and stretches. It's a visible sign of the coordination and strength your baby is developing. The increased size and weight can bring about some physical discomforts for her, such as back pain or balance changes. It's important to support her through these shifts by encouraging gentle exercises and ensuring she has comfortable seating. These alterations in her body reflect the baby's incredible progress and are a testament to the life growing within.

To better understand these developments, try asking your healthcare provider to use tools like 3D ultrasound imagery. These images give you a sneak peek into the womb, allowing you to visualize the baby's form and movements.

Building a stronger team during pregnancy

The second trimester offers a unique opportunity to strengthen your bond with your wife or partner as you both adjust to the reality that a new family member is on the way. It's a time to focus on strengthening your relationship—for your benefit but also the future well-being of your baby. One of the most effective ways to reinforce your connection is by participating in couples' prenatal classes. These classes are educational and also, they provide a shared experience that can bring you closer together. You'll learn about labor, delivery, and newborn care while gaining practical insights into supporting each other during the Big Day. It's a chance to practice teamwork, and you'll meet other expectant parents navigating the same uncertainties and joys.

Regular, intentional date nights are another great way to keep the spark alive. Now, these don't have to be elaborate or expensive. It's the quality time spent together that counts. Try cooking a meal together at home or taking a stroll in the park. These moments of connection will remind you of the partnership that started this adventure. Amidst the excitement and planning for the baby's arrival, it can be easy to lose sight of each other as individuals. Date nights offer a chance to step back from the preparation frenzy and simply enjoy each other's company.

Intimacy during pregnancy can be a sensitive topic, but it's important for maintaining both physical and emotional closeness. She needs to know that you still find her attractive and desirable so be sure to tell her this. As long as there are no complications, sexual relations can continue as usual. However, it's perfectly normal for intimacy to shift as her body changes. You may need to try new things – have fun and keep your sense of humor! The main thing is to keep the lines of communication open, discussing what feels comfortable and what doesn't. Small moves, like kicking back on the couch together or giving each other a massage can be wonderful. These small acts of affection can go a long way in affirming your love and care for each other, even if traditional forms of intimacy need to be adjusted.

Talk about how you envision your roles as parents and any concerns you might have. These conversations lay the groundwork for a collaborative parenting approach, ensuring that you're aligned in your expectations and ready to support each other as you grow into your roles as Mom and Dad.

Showing up for training camp: Getting engaged in prenatal appointments and classes

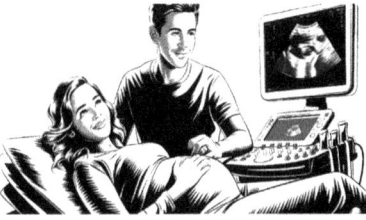

Walking into a prenatal appointment can feel a bit daunting as it's like stepping into the heart of the pregnancy experience. You enter a room filled with anticipation, where each visit unveils new insights about your growing baby. As an expectant dad, actively participating in these appointments is incredibly beneficial for both of you. It's a chance to witness your baby's progress firsthand, reinforcing the reality of what's to come.

During these visits, healthcare professionals will conduct various procedures designed to ensure the pregnancy progresses smoothly. You'll encounter the anatomy scan, a detailed ultrasound that checks the baby's physical development. During this scan, you might catch a glimpse of your baby's tiny fingers and toes and perhaps even discover the baby's sex. Monitoring fetal growth is a regular part of these check-ups, ensuring everything is on track.

Prenatal classes are another essential component of preparing for parenthood. These classes are like an all-star playbook of knowledge, offering invaluable skills and insights as the due date approaches. You'll learn about birthing techniques, which can simplify labor, making it less intimidating. Understanding what to expect during labor can help you support her more effectively, ensuring you're both on the same page when the big day arrives. Things like how to know when to drive your wife to the hospital, what to take with you, and how to support her will be explained. Newborn care basics are also covered, equipping you with practical skills like diapering and bathing, which can boost your confidence as a new dad. These classes often generate a sense of community, connecting you with other couples on a similar path. Many couples make a few friends at these classes and keep in touch with each other after the birth.

Building a relationship with healthcare providers is an often overlooked but important aspect of prenatal care. These professionals are not just there to guide you through medical procedures; they are allies in your parenthood journey. Openly engaging with them can lead to a more personalized and supportive experience. Don't ever hesitate to ask questions, no matter how small they might seem. Communicating with your healthcare provider ensures that you're informed and prepared, whether it's about your partner's health, the baby's development, or your personal concerns. This collaborative approach creates a partnership where both parties work together to ensure the best outcomes for both mom and baby. You'll feel more supported and confident in the care you both receive, knowing that you have an expert team ready to assist and guide you through every stage.

Playing through the pressure: Tackling expectations and peer challenges

Becoming a dad can sometimes feel like stepping into a spotlight you didn't ask for. Society has a way of placing a heavy load of expectations on new fathers, often without the necessary support to back it up. You might feel the pressure to be the perfect provider, the all-knowing parent, and the supportive partner while maintaining a stoic front. Family members might offer unsolicited advice, question your parenting decisions, or compare you to other dads. Friends might joke about your impending lack of sleep or how your social life will vanish. While these pressures are often well-intentioned, they can weigh heavily on you, creating anxiety about whether you're measuring up.

Handling these pressures starts with staying true to your values and goals. You must remember that every family is unique, and what works for one might not work for another. Reflect on what kind of father you want to be and use that as your compass. When faced with criticism or advice that doesn't align with your beliefs, it's okay to politely acknowledge it and move on. Setting boundaries is vital. Let people know that while you appreciate their input, you and your partner are finding your own way. Sometimes, all it takes is a simple, "Thanks, we'll think about it" to deflect pressure without offending. It's helpful to have a mentor – perhaps an older man you admire with a successful marriage and whose kids have grown up into well-balanced, great people—to get advice from rather than trying to listen to her mother and your Aunt Mary and the guy you met at the office who has twins.

Open dialogues are helpful when dealing with societal norms and expectations. Discussing your feelings about external pressures can bring you closer and help you present a united front. Decide what values are most important to you as a family and how you plan to uphold them. This mutual understanding can make it easier to brush off outside comments and focus on what truly matters to you both. By sharing your concerns and discussing potential scenarios, you can strategize how to handle them. Knowing you're not alone and she has your back is reassuring.

I remember a conversation with a fellow dad who felt overwhelmed by his family's constant comparisons to his brother, who seemed to have parenting down to an art. He shared how he felt inadequate and stressed, trying to live up to an impossible standard. However, through open discussions with his wife, they created a plan to handle family gatherings and conversations. They focused on their strengths and celebrated their own milestones, which helped build his confidence. Hearing his story reminded me of the power of partnership and the importance of creating your own personal game plan.

Getting game-ready: Preparing for the physical changes ahead

As your wife or partner moves deeper into the second trimester, her body becomes a marvel of transformation. The changes are as beautiful as they are significant, with her belly growing more pronounced, a visible testament to the life within. You might notice her posture shifting to accommodate this change, and her center of gravity adjusts with it. Her skin may stretch, leading to itchiness, while her breasts continue to prepare for breastfeeding, becoming fuller and possibly more tender. These physical shifts are a natural part of pregnancy but can also bring discomfort and self-consciousness.

You can play a clutch role in helping her adapt to these physical changes, starting with her wardrobe. To lift her spirits, offer her an all-paid shopping trip for maternity clothes. Comfort becomes key as her body continues to change. Another area where your support is invaluable is in helping with mobility adjustments. Simple acts like offering a hand to help her up from a low seat or reaching for items on high shelves can prevent unnecessary strain.

As these physical changes unfold, they inevitably impact daily life. Tasks that once seemed trivial, like tying shoes or getting in and out of the car, require more effort and planning. Her energy levels might fluctuate, and specific activities could become more challenging as the pregnancy progresses. This is a time to reassess routines and delegate or modify tasks to suit her current needs. For instance, consider lowering the height of frequently used items in the kitchen or bathroom to reduce over-stretching. This period is also an excellent opportunity to embrace and practice patience, allowing her the time and space to adjust her pace.

Beyond the physical adjustments, it's important to prepare yourself for the emotional changes she will face. Pregnancy brings a rollercoaster of emotions, from excitement to vulnerability. She might feel self-conscious about her changing body or anxious about the responsibilities ahead. Being there for her emotionally is essential. Practically, you can offer reassurance that you know she'll be a great mom. Remind her of times you've seen her being good with kids. Assure her that she's got an excellent medical and support team on her side. Remind her that you'll be with her every step of the way. Validate her experiences and remind her of the incredible work her body is doing. Sometimes, she just needs to hear that she's beautiful and doing a fantastic job. These affirmations can strengthen her confidence and help her embrace the changes with grace.

Second trimester highlights: Key milestones to watch for

As she progresses through the second trimester, the baby inside her is undergoing remarkable transformations. Imagine a tiny being, slightly smaller than the size of a volleyball, nestled in her belly, roughly 9 ½ inches in diameter and weighing about 32 oz. This period marks a time of significant growth as your baby develops distinct physical features that bring the reality of parenthood closer to home. Their once translucent skin is thickening, the bones become more solid, and the baby's shape becomes more defined. This development is fascinating and a testament to the complexity and wonder of human growth.

The baby's major organ systems continue to mature, setting the stage for life outside the womb. The nervous system is firing up, connecting the brain to the rest of the body. This connection allows the baby to process signals and respond to the outside world. The lungs, though not yet in use, are practicing the motions of breathing, preparing for their debut after birth. The digestive system is also gearing up, with the baby swallowing amniotic fluid—a practice fundamental for developing the gut. Each of these developments is a small miracle, reflecting the intricate work happening within your partner's body.

Your baby's sensory world is coming alive as well. Around this time, the baby begins to hear, making your voice a comforting presence. Don't feel weird if you find yourself talking to the baby and feel connected as you imagine them listening. Touch is another sense that's awakening, with the baby feeling the confines of the womb and responding to subtle movements. The baby's movements become stronger and more noticeable. Your wife or partner might experience these as little flutters or kicks, especially as the baby stretches and explores their expanding environment.

All these physical changes are significant for the baby and mean a lot for you and your partner. The movements remind us of the life growing inside, turning what once seemed abstract into tangible reality. When you feel those kicks, it's the perfect time to start thinking about the kind of parent you want to be and how to prepare for the exciting but challenging months ahead.

So, with the second trimester wrapping up, you're moving closer to meeting your new teammate. The groundwork laid during these weeks sets the stage for the final trimester, where anticipation builds, and preparations take on new urgency.

3

The Home Stretch – Tackling the Third Trimester

You're relaxing at a coffee shop, recharging and taking a moment to pause, when you overhear a couple at the next table talking about their baby's upcoming arrival. The woman laughs about her frequent trips to the bathroom, and the man looks both puzzled and amazed. You can't help but smile, feeling a sense of connection with this soon-to-be dad. The third trimester is when the reality of parenthood truly sets in. It's the final stretch, full of excitement, anticipation, and plenty of challenges.

Third quarter game plan: What to expect in the final stretch

As you enter this last trimester, you'll notice your wife's body undergoing profound changes. Fatigue often returns with a vengeance, making even the easiest tasks feel like she's grinding through overtime. It's common for her to experience increased discomfort as her growing belly places extra strain on her back and joints. Frequent urination becomes the norm, thanks to the baby taking up valuable space in her abdomen. Then there are the Braxton Hicks contractions, those "practice" contractions that can catch you both off guard. These are normal, but it's a good idea to familiarize yourself with how they feel, as they can sometimes be mistaken for the real thing. Real contractions are regular, more frequent intervals with increased intensity. Braxton Hicks contractions tend to be irregular and go away with rest or a change of position.

With the due date approaching, it's natural for both of you to have concerns about labor and delivery. You might find yourselves lying awake at night, wondering if you're ready for the Big Day. *Will you recognize the signs of labor in time? Can you handle the intensity of the delivery room?* These anxieties are part of the package and acknowledging them is the first step in managing them.

Monitoring health becomes a top priority in these final weeks. Regular check-ups are vital for keeping track of both the baby's and your wife's well-being. Be vigilant about any warning signs, such as sudden swelling of the feet and ankles or severe headaches, which could indicate conditions like pre-eclampsia (a type of dangerously high blood pressure). Familiarize yourself with these symptoms and discuss them with your healthcare provider to know when to seek medical attention. Additionally, pay attention to the baby's movements. Is the baby kicking regularly? Any noticeable decrease in activity warrants a call to the doctor, as it could signify a need for closer monitoring. These steps, while simple, ensure that both mom and baby receive the care they need as the big day draws near.

Create a checklist of key health aspects to monitor during the third trimester. Include prompts for tracking fetal movements, recognizing signs of pre-eclampsia, and noting regular check-up schedules. You'll find this type of checklist really helpful as it will help you stay organized and proactive in ensuring your partner's well-being. Keep it visible on the fridge or in a shared digital document, allowing both of you to contribute and discuss any concerns as they arise. This collaborative approach will enhance your preparedness and reinforce your role as an active, involved partner during this critical phase. Below is a general third-trimester checklist to use as a guide:

Third Trimester Health Checklist

1. Fetal Movements

- **Daily Kick Counts**
  - **What to monitor:** Aim to feel at least 10 movements (kicks, flutters, rolls) over a 2-hour period.
  - **Prompt:** Note if there is a significant decrease in fetal movements or if your partner goes longer than usual without feeling the baby move.
  - **Action:** If you notice reduced activity, encourage her to drink some water or juice, lie down quietly, and count again. If still low, contact your healthcare provider.

---

2. Blood Pressure & Signs of Pre-Eclampsia

- **Blood Pressure**
  - **What to monitor:** Track your partner's blood pressure if recommended by her healthcare provider (often via a home blood pressure monitor).
  - **Prompt:** Notify your doctor if her systolic (top number) is 140 or higher, or if her diastolic (bottom number) is 90 or higher.

- **Signs of Pre-Eclampsia**
  - **What to watch for:**
    - Persistent headache
    - Visual disturbances (blurring, flashing lights)
    - Sudden or severe swelling of hands, feet, or face
    - Pain in the upper right abdomen (under ribs)
    - Nausea or vomiting in late pregnancy
  - **Action:** Immediately call your healthcare provider or go to the hospital if your partner experiences any of these symptoms.

3. Regular Prenatal Check-Ups

- **Frequency**
  - **Weeks 28-36: Typically every 2 weeks** (depending on your provider's recommendation).
  - **Weeks 36-40 (or delivery):** Weekly visits.

- **Key Check-Up Components**
    - **Fundal Height & Baby's Position:** To assess fetal growth and position (head-down vs. breech).
    - **Heart Rate Monitoring:** Doppler or NST (Non-Stress Test) to check Baby's heart rate.
    - **Weight and Urine Checks:** Monitoring for protein in urine and significant or sudden weight changes.
    - **Blood Tests (If Needed):** To track iron levels, glucose levels (especially if your partner has gestational diabetes), and other markers.

4. Contractions and Preterm Labor Signs

- **What to monitor:**
    - **Frequency & Pattern of Contractions:** Are they coming at regular intervals, or do they subside when she rests or hydrates?
    - **Intensity:** Painful or mild?
    - **Any Leakage of Fluid or Bleeding:** Could signal rupture of membranes or other concerns.
- **Action**: If you notice more than six contractions in an hour before 37 weeks, or any fluid leakage or bleeding, contact your healthcare provider immediately.

5. General Wellness Checks

- **Swelling & Edema -** Mild swelling in feet and ankles can be normal; however, watch for sudden swelling in hands or face.
- **Sleep & Rest -** Use pillows for support; note if insomnia or discomfort worsens (possibly due to restless legs, frequent urination, or heartburn).
- **Nutrition & Hydration**
    - Keep a balanced diet rich in protein, fiber, vitamins, and minerals.
    - Ensure your partner stays hydrated; aim for 8–10 glasses of water a day (adjust based on climate and activity level).
- **Emotional Well-Being**
    - Monitor her mood, stress, and anxiety levels.
    - If she's feeling overwhelmed or persistently low, reach out to a counselor, support group, or your healthcare provider.

6. Additional Concerns & Reminders

- **Kick Count Log:** Keep a simple chart (paper or an app) to track fetal movements daily.
- **Blood Pressure Log:** If advised, note readings at the same time each day.
- **Hospital Bag Prep:** Aim to have a hospital bag ready by weeks 36-37. Include personal items, baby clothes, and important documents.
- **Birth Plan Review:** Discuss your preferences with your healthcare provider and birth partner.
- **Pediatrician Selection:** If you haven't already, consider choosing a pediatrician and scheduling an initial consultation.

7. When to Call Your Healthcare Provider Immediately

1. **Decreased or No Fetal Movement** despite your usual tactics (drinking something cold/sweet and lying down).
2. **Possible Signs of Labor** before 37 weeks: regular contractions, leaking fluid, or bloody show.
3. **Symptoms of Pre-Eclampsia:** Severe headache, vision changes, or upper abdominal pain.
4. **High Blood Pressure Readings** above the thresholds recommended by your doctor.
5. **Any Other Unusual Concerns** that cause worry or discomfort.

Third-trimester training camp: Breaking down your baby's progress

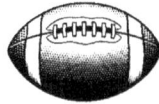

As you enter the third trimester, your baby is making remarkable strides in development. Your baby is about as long as a football at 28 weeks and can now open their eyes. It's in this trimester that the brain and vision undergo rapid development, setting the stage for those wide-eyed first moments after birth. By the time you reach the 30-week mark, your baby measures about 16 inches long and responds to light by opening and closing their eyes—a fascinating peek into their growing awareness of the outside world. The lungs, too, are working hard, practicing breathing rhythms that will be vital once the baby is born. This period of growth is necessary for maturing organs and establishing regular sleep patterns, which might explain why you notice more periods of quiet than activity. The immune system gains strength, better preparing the baby to handle life outside the womb.

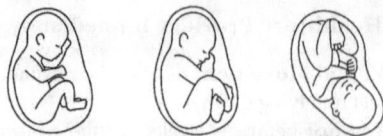

As the weeks pass, your baby begins serious preparations for the journey ahead. By the time you reach the 33rd week, the baby is roughly 4 pounds and actively practicing swallowing, yawning, and even breathing movements. Their brain now plays a significant role in regulating body temperature—a skill they'll need soon. Around this time, your baby should start positioning themselves head-down, a natural alignment for birth. This head-down position is important, as it aligns the baby for the safest possible delivery. They also start accumulating fat, giving their skin a healthy, pink hue and helping regulate body temperature once they are no longer snug in the womb.

Bonding with your unborn baby during this time can be a comforting and rewarding experience. Talking and singing to the baby can be a simple yet powerful way to make a connection. Your voice is a familiar sound they've been hearing for months, and it's known to have a calming effect. When you feel those kicks, take a moment to respond, even if it's just a gentle press against your partner's belly. It's a unique form of communication that can strengthen your bond. These interactions aren't just for fun; they can actually stimulate the baby's developing senses and promote a sense of security.

Game day prep: Planning for the big moment

As the third trimester unfolds, it's time to dive into the practicalities of delivery planning. Choosing a birthing location is one of the first decisions you'll face. Whether it's a hospital, a birthing center, or even a home birth, each option has its merits, depending on your preferences and circumstances. Visit potential locations together, ask questions, and get a feel for the environment. Consider the distance from home, the amenities offered, the costs, and the level of medical support available. Once you've made your choice, understanding the location's protocols becomes essential. Get familiar with the admission process, visiting hours, and what's included in the postpartum care package. This knowledge will help reduce any last-minute surprises and ensure you're both comfortable with the setting.

Pain management is another critical aspect of delivery planning. The options range from medical interventions to natural methods, each with its own set of benefits. Epidural anesthesia is a popular choice for its effectiveness in numbing pain from the waist down, allowing her to remain awake and alert during childbirth. However, it's not for everyone, and some may prefer less invasive techniques. Natural pain relief methods, such as breathing exercises, massage, and hydrotherapy, can also be effective. Discuss these options with your partner and healthcare team to make informed decisions that align with her comfort level and birth plan. Knowing what's available can empower your wife or partner to make choices that feel right for her.

Your role as a birth partner is essential. Think of yourself as the coach of a three-on-three basketball team, there to advocate for your wife's wishes. This might mean communicating her preferences to medical staff or ensuring the environment is as she envisioned. Providing physical support, like offering a hand to squeeze or applying pressure to relieve back pain, can also be invaluable. Emotional support is just as crucial. Encourage her, remind her of her strength, and reassure her when doubts creep in. Your presence can be a source of immense comfort, helping her confidently surf the intense waves of labor.

Speaking of labor, recognizing its signs is also a top priority. Look for indicators like regular contractions, water breaking, and back pain. Knowing when to head to the hospital can prevent a mad dash in the middle of the night.

Preparation for the unexpected is another key element of delivery planning. Labor can be unpredictable, and it's wise to be ready for potential complications. An emergency C-section, for instance, might become necessary if the baby's health is at risk. Familiarize yourself with the procedure so you're not caught off guard. Remember, flexibility is your best friend during this time. While you can plan meticulously, staying open to changes ensures you're equipped to handle whatever comes your way.

Staying in the zone: Handling emotional and physical stress

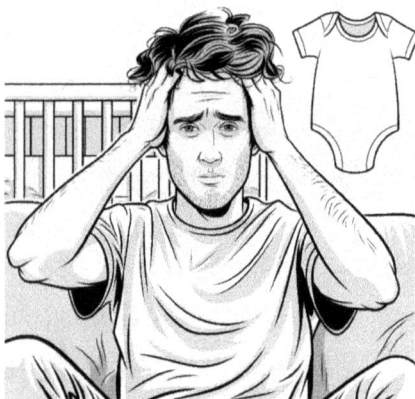

As the third trimester progresses, the weight of anticipation can bring its own set of stressors. The fear of labor and delivery often looms large, creating a sense of anxiety that can be hard to shake. You might find yourself juggling work commitments while trying to be present for your wife, feeling like you're being pulled in all directions. I've been there. This balancing act between professional duties and personal responsibilities can be taxing. It's common to feel overwhelmed as you both prepare for the life-changing event just around the corner. Recognizing these stressors is essential, as they can impact your partner's well-being and the harmony of your relationship. It's a pivotal time when emotional support and open communication become your best assets.

Think about adding stress management techniques into your daily routine to alleviate the pressure. Practicing mindfulness can be incredibly beneficial, helping you stay grounded amidst the chaos. Exercises like deep breathing or meditation can offer a moment of peace, allowing you to step back and refocus. Light physical activities, such as a leisurely walk or mild stretches, can also help release tension. These activities improve your physical health and provide an opportunity for both of you to connect and share in a calming experience. Encouraging each other to engage in these practices can create a supportive environment where stress is managed jointly.

Open discussions about fears and anxieties are important during this stage. Set aside time to discuss the concerns weighing on each of your minds. Whether it's the logistics of delivery or worries about adjusting to parenthood, voicing these thoughts can be liberating. These conversations allow you to address fears head-on and find solutions together. It's important to listen actively, providing reassurance and understanding. By promoting an atmosphere of honesty, you build a foundation of trust that will serve you well in the challenging yet rewarding days ahead.

Amidst the mad scramble of preparations, don't forget the importance of self-care. As a dad-to-be, your mental and physical health is just as important as your partner and baby's. Set aside personal time to recharge, whether it's catching up on a hobby, exercising, or simply enjoying a quiet moment alone. This recharge is vital for maintaining your energy and patience. Seeking support from friends and family can also provide a necessary outlet. Whether sharing your experiences with fellow dads or leaning on loved ones for advice, having a support network can make a significant difference. Embrace these connections, knowing that caring for yourself ultimately benefits your partner and future child.

Mastering the mental game: Building patience and understanding

As you count down the days to the arrival of your new baby, patience becomes an invaluable ally. The final stretch of pregnancy can feel like the longest overtime of your life, and the waiting game might start to test your resolve. Yet, patience is crucial now more than ever. The due date may be circled on your calendar, but babies have their own schedules and sometimes take their sweet time. This period requires a gentle reminder to yourself that the wait is not just about anticipation but also preparation. Each day brings your baby closer to being ready for the world, and your wife or partner needs your steady, patient presence as her body undergoes the last stages of this incredible transformation.

Setting realistic expectations is key to maintaining patience. Understand that things might not go exactly as planned, but that's perfectly okay. Life with a baby is unpredictable, so embrace flexibility. Creating a flexible schedule allows you to adapt to sudden changes without feeling overwhelmed. If plans need to shift or tasks take longer than expected, remind yourself that these are just part of the process. This mindset can alleviate anxiety and keep you calm and supportive. A flexible approach helps you be more present and focused on what truly matters—being there for your wife or partner.

Understanding her needs during this time is also paramount. Her body and mood might fluctuate, and being attuned to these changes can make a significant difference. Offering reassurance and encouragement can provide her with the comfort she needs. Sometimes, a simple "You're doing great" can lift her spirits. Pay attention to her cues and adapt to her changing moods. Some days, she might need a quiet moment to herself, while on others, she might seek your company. Be her ally, ready to support her in whatever way she needs. This understanding creates a sense of security and partnership, reinforcing your commitment to this shared experience.

Empathy and compassion should be at the forefront of every interaction. You're both in the final stretch of the game, going up against an opponent you've never faced before, so a supportive and nurturing environment is essential. Approach each situation with empathy, putting yourself in her shoes to understand her perspective. Compassion goes a long way in creating a supportive atmosphere where both partners feel valued and understood. It strengthens your bond, paving the way for a harmonious transition into parenthood. Through empathy, you support your partner and prepare yourself for the compassionate, caring dad you aspire to be.

Third quarter recap: Key milestones

As you approach the finish line of the third trimester, it's incredible to realize just how much your baby has grown. Weighing in at about 7.5 pounds and measuring roughly 20 inches long, your baby has been on quite the growth spurt. This rapid growth is essential, as the baby builds up fat reserves to help regulate body temperature once they're out in the big world. It's like watching a tiny miracle unfold, knowing that each ounce gained is preparing your little one for their grand debut. These last few weeks are vital for development, making every moment count as the baby readies themselves for life outside the womb.

Inside, the baby is working hard to put the finishing touches on their organs. The brain is firing on all cylinders, establishing the neural connections that will support everything from basic functions to cognitive development. Meanwhile, the lungs are practicing the motions of breathing, ensuring they're ready for that first cry. The immune system also gears up, building the defenses needed to fend off the dangers in the outside world. This organ maturation is vital, laying the groundwork for a healthy start. It's fascinating to think about how this tiny being is getting ready to navigate a new environment, equipped with the essentials for survival.

Sensory development is another exciting aspect of the third trimester. Your baby can now see, hear, taste, and respond to touch. They might even recognize the sound of your voice or the rhythm of your movements. These sensory experiences prepare the baby for the sensory-rich world they're about to enter. Imagine your baby getting used to the feel of your gentle touch, the sound of your favorite tunes, or the taste of amniotic fluid, which will soon be replaced by breast milk or formula. These developments are a testament to the complexity and wonder of human growth and a reminder of the intricate processes that occur even before birth.

As the baby prepares for birth, they usually naturally shift into a head-down position, aligning themselves for the journey through the birth canal. This shift clearly signals that they're getting ready to meet you. It's a time of tremendous anticipation, knowing that soon enough, you'll be holding this tiny person in your arms.

With your baby almost ready to join the world, the pregnancy is about to come to an end. You've tackled the complexities of the third trimester, from physical growth to sensory development, with each passing day bringing you closer to meeting your baby. As you prepare for the new chapter of life outside the womb, embrace the anticipation and excitement of what's to come. Your baby is nearly ready, and so are you. Your parenthood adventure is just beginning!

4

Game Day Strategy – Prepping for Your Baby's Big Arrival

T he anticipation of welcoming your newborn is a feeling unlike any other. I remember standing in the nursery, folding tiny onesies, and wondering how our lives were about to change. But amidst all the excitement, a little voice whispered, "Are you ready?" You're not alone if you've ever found yourself in a similar moment. Preparing for your baby's arrival can be as overwhelming as it is exhilarating, and a key part of this preparation is creating a birth plan with your wife or partner. A birth plan will help you feel more in control, manage your expectations, and ease some anxiety. It's a written document outlining your labor and delivery preferences, offering a sense of control and inclusion in decision-making. Think of it as your opportunity to take an active role in the birth experience, ensuring your wishes are known and respected.

The birth plan

Creating a birth plan starts with open and honest conversations with your wife. Sit down together and discuss what matters most to each of you. What kind of birth experience do you envision? Do you have specific preferences for pain relief or labor positions? Understanding hospital protocols

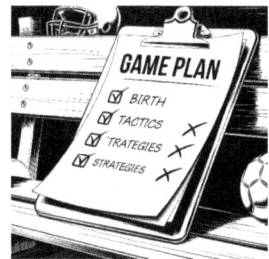

is important here. Visit the hospital beforehand to familiarize yourselves with the setting and procedures. Ask questions about labor and delivery practices, and gather information on what's available. You'll want to know about the availability of birthing rooms, the use of medical interventions, and how the hospital handles unexpected situations. This knowledge can provide reassurance and help both of you feel more prepared.

When drafting your birth plan, respect your partner's preferences for pain relief. Some may opt for natural methods like breathing exercises or hydrotherapy, while others might prefer an epidural. Discuss these options together, weighing the pros and cons of each, and make sure to communicate your choices to your healthcare provider. Deciding on the presence of support people is something else to decide on. Some couples prefer an intimate setting with just the two of them, while others welcome family members or a doula for additional support. A doula is a trained professional who provides physical, emotional, and informational support to individuals before, during, and after childbirth. Doulas do not provide medical care but offer guidance, comfort measures, and advocacy to help parents have a more positive birthing experience. Whatever you choose, ensure it aligns with what makes both of you feel most comfortable and supported.

Flexibility is key when it comes to birth plans. While having a plan is important, it's essential to remain adaptable to changing circumstances. Labor can be unpredictable, and unforeseen medical interventions may become necessary for the health of the mother or baby. This is where the power of flexibility comes into play. Being open to adjustments ensures you're prepared for whatever may arise without feeling like you've lost control. Remember, the ultimate goal is a healthy baby and mom, so trust in the expertise of your healthcare team and be ready to pivot if needed.

Collaboration with healthcare providers is essential. Share your birth plan with them well before the due date, allowing ample time for discussion and alignment. This collaboration ensures that your preferences are understood and respected while accommodating any medical requirements. Establishing a good rapport with your healthcare team can enhance communication and make the labor and delivery process smoother. They're there to support you, and having a clear understanding of your plan helps them provide the best care possible.

You may want to use a birth plan worksheet to organize your thoughts and preferences. This can be helpful when discussing options with your partner and healthcare provider. Include sections for pain relief preferences, labor positions, and any special requests for the delivery room environment. This worksheet can be a central resource for your birth plan discussions, ensuring all key topics are covered and documented. Below is a birth plan worksheet from the American College of Obstetricians and Gynecologists (ACOG).

Birth Plan Worksheet

Personal Information:

Name: _____

Partner/Support Person: _____

Due Date: _____

Doctor/Midwife: _____

Hospital/Birth Center: _____

Emergency Contact: _____

Labor Preferences:

1. **Environment:**
   - Dim lighting
   - Music/playlist (preferred genre: _____)
   - Minimal noise
   - Aromatherapy (specific scents: _____)
   - Other: _____

2. **Support Team:**
   - Partner
   - Doula
   - Family member(s) (specify: _____)
   - Friend(s)
   - Other: _____
3. **Pain Management:**
   - Natural methods (breathing, massage, movement)
   - Epidural
   - IV pain medication
   - TENS unit
   - Other: _____
   - Preferences regarding timing: _____
4. **Positions for Labor and Delivery:**
   - Walking
   - Squatting
   - Using a birthing ball
   - Lying on side
   - Water birth (if available)
   - Other: _____
5. **Monitoring Preferences:**
   - Intermittent monitoring
   - Continuous monitoring
   - Wireless monitoring (if available)
   - Other: _____

Delivery Preferences:

1. **Pushing:**
   - Spontaneous pushing
   - Directed pushing
   - Use of mirror to see progress
   - Other: _____
2. **Episiotomy:**
   - Prefer to avoid unless medically necessary

   - Open to discussion
   - Other: _____
3. **Delivery Assistance:**
   - Prefer natural delivery
   - Open to vacuum/forceps assistance if needed
4. **Other:** _____
5. **Cord Cutting:**
   - Partner/support person to cut the cord
   - Delayed cord clamping
   - Other: _____

Post-Birth Preferences:

1. **Skin-to-Skin Contact:**
   - Immediate skin-to-skin after birth
   - Partner/support person to hold Baby if I'm unable
2. **Feeding Preferences:**
   - Breastfeeding
   - Formula feeding
   - Combination
   - Other: _____
3. **Newborn Care:**
   - Delay initial bath
   - Administer Vitamin K shot
   - Administer eye ointment
   - Other: _____
4. **Rooming-In:**
   - Baby stays with me at all times
   - Open to nursery care as needed

Unexpected Circumstances:

1. **Cesarean Section (if necessary):**
   - Partner/support person present
   - Skin-to-skin in operating room
   - Breastfeeding in recovery room
   - Other: _____

2. **If Baby Requires Special Care:**
   - Partner/support person accompanies Baby
   - I would like to visit the NICU as soon as possible
   - Other: _____

Another great reference for a more detailed and customizable birth plan can be found on TheBump.com (https://www.thebump.com/a/tool-bir th-plan#3).

Preparing the turf: Essential nursery prep tips

Transforming a room into a nursery is one of those defining tasks that makes the impending arrival of your newborn feel more real. It's an opportunity to create a functional and welcoming space where your baby will spend countless hours sleeping, playing, and growing. Start with the crib, the centerpiece of any nursery. Ensure it's safe by using a crib manufactured after 2011, meeting the latest safety standards. The crib mattress should be firm and locked in without gaps to reduce the risk of suffocation. Steer clear of pillows, blankets, and stuffed animals in the crib to minimize hazards. The changing station is another important area. Position it within easy reach of diapers, wipes, and creams. Think about adding shelves or drawers to keep supplies organized and easily accessible. This setup makes diaper changes smoother and keeps the nursery tidy.

Safety is paramount, so consider securing furniture to the walls to prevent tipping accidents. Babies are naturally curious, and they don't take long to start pulling themselves up. Anchoring bookshelves and dressers adds an extra layer of protection. Installing a baby monitor can also offer peace of mind, allowing you to keep an eye on your baby from any room in the house. Choose a monitor with clear video and sound quality for the best results. As you plan the nursery layout, ensure that cords, outlets, and other potential hazards are out of reach. Cover electrical outlets and tuck cords away to prevent curious hands from exploring them. These precautions help create a safe environment where your baby can explore with minimal risk.

Comfort and practicality go hand in hand when designing a nursery that works for you and your baby. Invest in a comfortable rocking chair or glider for feeding and bonding. You'll spend many nights here, so choose something that supports your back and arms. Adequate lighting is important, too. Install a dimmer switch with adjustable brightness levels to create a soothing atmosphere for nighttime feeds. This helps ease the transition between sleep and wakefulness, keeping your baby calm and relaxed. Look for storage solutions that make finding clothes, blankets, and toys easy. Baskets, bins, and drawer organizers can keep everything in its place, reducing clutter and simplifying daily routines.

Adding personal touches is the fun part that transforms the nursery from a bare room into a space that feels like home. Incorporate family

photos or cherished mementos to create a sense of connection and be-
longing. These items serve as visual reminders of the love that surrounds
your baby. Choose a soothing color scheme, like soft pastels or calming
neutrals, to promote relaxation and warmth. You may want to add a mural
or wall decals that reflect your family's personality and interests, whether
it's a beach scene or a starry night sky. These personal elements make the
nursery uniquely yours; a special place where your baby will feel cherished
and secure.

Defending the stadium: Baby-proofing essentials

When you're getting ready to welcome a newborn, baby-proofing is one of
those tasks that might not seem urgent at first. Still, it's essential for your
baby's safety and your peace of mind. Before you know it, your little one
will be crawling, exploring, and getting into everything they can reach. The
best time to start baby-proofing is during pregnancy, ideally in the second
trimester when you have the energy and time to tackle this important job.
You'll want to ensure that your home is a safe haven, free from potential
hazards that curious hands might find.

Start by conducting a hazard assessment throughout your home. Walk
through each room, looking for anything that could pose a risk. Identify
sharp edges, unsecured furniture, or small objects that could be choking
hazards. Declutter spaces where items might be within reach of a crawling
baby. This initial assessment will give you a clear picture of what must be
addressed.

In common areas like the living room, safety is a priority. Secure furniture, such as bookcases and television stands, to the walls to prevent them
from tipping over. These heavy items can be particularly dangerous once
your baby starts pulling themselves up. Floor safety is another consideration. Ensure rugs have non-slip pads underneath to prevent slips and falls.
Electrical cords and outlets should be out of reach and covered with safety

plugs. These measures can mitigate risks and create a safer environment for your child to explore.

In the kitchen, focus on appliance safety and cabinet security. Install safety latches on cabinets containing cleaning supplies or sharp objects. Keep trash cans covered or out of reach to prevent curious hands from sifting through them. Cooking can pose a risk as well; use stove knob covers and get into the habit now of turning pot handles inward to prevent burns. These adjustments might take some getting used to, but they significantly reduce the chances of accidents.

If you have pets, preparing them for the arrival of a baby is critical. While mom and baby are still in the hospital, introduce them to the baby's scent using blankets or clothing. This familiarization can help ease the transition and prevent anxiety when the baby comes home. Teaching pets your boundaries is vital, such as avoiding the nursery, crib, or baby's play area when you are not around. This training can ensure a harmonious relationship between your pets and the newest family member.

Additional precautions are necessary in stairs and hallways. Install baby gates at the top and bottom of the stairs. These gates should be securely mounted and easy for adults to operate but difficult for little ones to maneuver. It's also wise to keep hallways clear of obstacles that might trip a toddler while they are taking their first steps.

Water safety and proper storage of medications and chemicals are top priorities in the bathroom. Never leave your baby unattended in the bath, even for a moment. Use non-slip mats in the tub and always ensure the water temperature is safe by pre-testing the water. Store medications and cleaning supplies out of reach, preferably in a locked cabinet. This precaution prevents accidental ingestion and keeps potentially harmful substances away from small hands. A little preparation now can avoid a lot of worry later, allowing you to stay in the zone and cherish every moment with your little champ.

Game day gear: The ultimate hospital bag checklist

When heading to the hospital for the delivery, having a well-packed bag for mom and baby can make all the difference. Typically, the mom will have everything in order well before her delivery date. However, suppose the baby decides to arrive unexpectedly early. In that case, you can step in and save the day by gathering the following simple necessities. For the mother, comfort is paramount. Pack a few sets of comfortable clothing that are easy to get on and off, such as loose-fitting tops and pants. Don't forget a cozy robe and a pair of slippers with a good grip for those first post-delivery steps. Toiletry essentials—think toothbrush, toothpaste, face wipes, shower gel, and deodorant—are a must. Remember to pack her hairbrush and comb. If she has long hair, a scrunchie to keep her hair back will be appreciated. Having her personal care items on hand can help her feel more at home in the hospital environment. She'll probably need some lip balm too. Don't forget about the birth plan we discussed earlier. Tuck a copy of it into the bag as well. While you might have discussed it with your healthcare provider, having it readily accessible will ensure everyone is on the same page. Ensure you also pack phone chargers, as friends and relatives will be blowing up your phones with texts and phone calls during your stay in the hospital.

Pack a few outfits for the baby's debut, including a going-home ensemble. Opt for soft, breathable fabrics that are gentle on newborn skin. A couple of blankets will come in handy for swaddling and keeping the baby cozy during the hospital stay. Plus, diapers, of course! Don't forget about the car seat—double-check that it's installed correctly in your vehicle ahead of time. This isn't just for practicality; it's a safety requirement for taking your baby home. Ensure it meets all current safety standards and that you and your partner know how to use it properly. The last thing you want on discharge day is to fumble with straps and buckles so have a practice session before the time.

As the dad, your time at the hospital can feel long without the right provisions. Bringing snacks and drinks will keep your energy up during labor and beyond. Hospitals have vending machines, but having your own stash means you won't have to leave her side when hunger strikes. Entertainment options are a lifesaver during downtime, so consider packing a book, tablet, or even a deck of cards. Whether it's a favorite movie or some music, these personal comforts can make the wait more pleasant. Keep your phone charger and digital camera handy to capture those first precious moments. You'll want to remember this time, and having the right tech tools ensures you won't miss a thing.

Preparing for the unexpected is a wise move. Labor can be unpredictable, and your stay might be longer than anticipated. Pack extra clothes for you and mom-to-be to accommodate an extended stay. Think of light layers, as hospital temperatures can fluctuate. Have all the necessary documents on hand, such as insurance information and personal identification. These items might seem an afterthought, but they're often needed at unexpected times. It's better to have them and not need them than to be caught off guard. When you're wrapped up in the excitement and nerves of the moment, being prepared can help keep stress at bay, allowing you to focus on what truly matters: welcoming your new baby into the world.

Below is a comprehensive checklist of items you may want to pack for the hospital or birthing center. You can adjust it based on personal preferences and what your hospital provides.

Ultimate Mom/Baby Hospital Bag Checklist

For Mom:

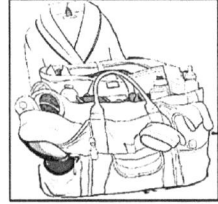

1. **Important Documents**
   - Photo ID (driver's license, passport)
   - Health insurance card
   - Hospital registration forms
   - Birth plan (several copies)
2. **Comfort and Labor Items**
   - Comfortable labor/delivery gown (hospital will provide one, but she may prefer her own)
   - Robe or cardigan
   - Warm socks or slippers with non-slip soles
   - Flip-flops (for the shower)
   - Pillow from home (in a distinct pillowcase)
   - Lip balm
   - Hair ties, headbands, or clips
   - Relaxation aids (e.g., essential oils, music, stress balls)
   - Phone/tablet, charger, earphones
3. **Toiletries**
   - Toothbrush and toothpaste
   - Hairbrush or comb
   - Shampoo and conditioner (travel-sized)
   - Face wash, moisturizer, makeup (if desired)
   - Deodorant
   - Contact lens solution, case, and glasses (if applicable)
   - Perineal spray or witch hazel pads (if preferred)

4. **Postpartum Essentials**
   - Nursing bras or sports bras
   - Breast pads (disposable or reusable)
   - Maternity pads or heavy-flow sanitary pads
   - Comfortable high-waisted underwear (big enough to hold large pads)
   - Nipple cream (if planning to breastfeed)
   - Loose, comfortable clothes for post-delivery
   - Sleepwear (button-down nightgown or pajamas for easy nursing)
5. **Going-Home Outfit**
   - Loose, comfortable clothing (consider maternity clothes)
   - Slip-on shoes

6. **Snacks and Hydration**
   - Healthy, energy-boosting snacks (e.g., granola bars, dried fruit, nuts)
   - Water bottle (with straw or spout)
   - Electrolyte drinks or coconut water

For Baby:
   - Newborn and 0–3-month onesies (2-3)
   - Sleepers (2-3)
   - Socks and mittens
   - Baby hat
   - Going-home outfit (weather-appropriate)
1. **Diapering**
   - Newborn diapers (hospital usually provides some, but extra can be helpful)
   - Unscented baby wipes
   - Diaper cream
2. **Blankets and Swaddles**
   - Swaddle blankets (hospital often provides these, but can bring your own)
   - Receiving blanket
3. **Car Seat**
   - Approved, rear-facing infant car seat installed in the car prior to discharge
4. **Feeding Items (if not breastfeeding)**
   - Formula (check with hospital on what they provide)
   - Bottles and nipples

For Partner/Support Person:
   - Phone and charger
   - Camera (optional) and batteries/memory card
   - Comfortable clothing for a couple of days
   - Toiletries (toothbrush, deodorant, etc.)
   - Snacks and drinks
   - Small pillow and light blanket (optional)
   - Cash or change for vending machines or parking

Extra Items:
   - A small amount of cash for any hospital-related fees or tips
   - Thank-you cards or a small treat for hospital staff (optional)
   - White noise machine or portable speaker (optional)
   - Extension cord for chargers (outlets may be far away)

Tips:
   - Check with your hospital or birth center to see what they provide (e.g., diapers, wipes, postpartum supplies).
   - Pack your bags several weeks before your due date.
   - Keep the car seat installed or ready for installation ahead of time.
   - Leave valuables and expensive jewelry at home.

This list can be customized based on your specific needs and your hospital's policies.

Starting strong: Managing the first days at home

When you first step through the front door with your newborn, life feels very different. It's both exhilarating and daunting as if you've just unlocked a new level in a video game you've never played. Going from the hospital's structured environment to an unpredictable home turf can be a shock, as nurses and doctors are no longer readily available for the hundreds of questions that instantly pop into your mind when you get home. Suddenly, you and your wife are in charge, and it's your decisions and actions that matter most. Coordinating with family and friends for support can ease this transition. Having loved ones ready to lend a hand can make the adjustment smoother—they can bring over a meal, run errands, or just be there for moral support. Capture those first family moments, too. They're fleeting; before you know it, your tiny bundle will be a bustling toddler. Taking photos or videos can preserve the memories of the day when you brought your baby home.

Settling into new routines is vital for everyone's sanity. Babies thrive on consistency, and establishing routines can help them—and you—adjust to the world outside the womb. Start by implementing a simple feeding schedule, sleeping, and wake time. As you observe your baby's natural rhythms, you'll see patterns emerge, which can guide you in adapting routines that fit your new family.

Emotional changes are part and parcel of bringing home a newborn. It's a roller coaster of feelings—joy, exhaustion, and everything in between. Recognizing signs of postpartum mood shifts in your wife or partner is vital. She might experience mood swings, anxiety, or even sadness, and it's important to address these feelings with empathy and support. Encourage open conversations about how she's feeling and remind her that it's okay to ask for help. Seeking support from family and friends can be invaluable—whether it's a listening ear or practical assistance. As for you, adjusting to your role as a new dad can bring emotional challenges. Embrace these changes, and remember that it's a shared experience and not perfect. You're both in this together, learning and growing as parents.

Building confidence in your parenting skills takes time, but trust your instincts. You're more capable than you might think. Celebrate the small successes, like mastering a diaper change or soothing your baby to sleep. These little victories will boost your confidence and reinforce your ability to care for your newborn. Embrace the learning process early on—mistakes are part of it, and each one teaches you something new. Remember, every parent was once in your shoes, feeling unsure and figuring things out. You're not alone, and with each passing day, you'll find your stride. It's about progress, not perfection, and creating a loving environment where your baby can thrive. Keep reminding yourself that you're doing a fantastic job, even when it feels challenging.

Building a winning routine with your new teammate

Your life as a new dad is like stepping onto the field for the first time, with every play yet to be called. Establishing a routine with your newborn is like building a solid game plan—it brings structure and keeps your days running smoothly. Routines offer a comforting rhythm in a time that can feel chaotic. They benefit both you and your baby by providing a sense of security and stability. Knowing what comes next—whether it's feeding time, a nap, or play—helps your little one feel safe in their new world. For you, routines can turn the unpredictable into the manageable, offering a playbook to navigate your new role as a father.

Creating a routine that works involves balancing consistency with flexibility. Babies, as you'll soon discover, have their own unique rhythms. Some may sleep soundly through the night early on, while others wake frequently for many months. The key is to build a schedule that accommodates these natural patterns. Start with the basics: feeding and nap times.

Newborns typically eat every few hours and sleep a lot—though often in short bursts. They have tiny stomachs, meaning they must feed often, sometimes every two to three hours. This can feel overwhelming, but it's a chance to bond during these quiet moments. Pay attention to your baby's cues and help your partner adjust the schedule accordingly. If they seem hungry before the next scheduled feeding, be flexible and feed them. Likewise, if they're still soundly sleeping when it's time to wake up, give them a little more time. This adaptability ensures that routines support rather than constrain your baby's needs. It's a learning process for parents and the baby, and flexibility is key. Don't be afraid to tweak things as you go. The routine that works today might need a little adjusting tomorrow, and that's perfectly normal.

Sharing responsibilities is essential to maintaining balance and team-work in this new chapter of life. Consider dividing nighttime duties so both of you get some rest. If mom isn't breastfeeding, assist by taking over some feedings to allow her to sleep. You could handle the mid-night feeds while your partner takes the early morning shift. Rotating feeding and diapering tasks can also prevent burnout and create a sense of shared responsibility. It's important to communicate openly about what works and what doesn't, adjusting roles as needed. Teamwork strengthens your partnership and creates a supportive environment for your baby, who benefits from the love and care of both parents.

As your baby grows, your established routines will need to evolve. Babies change quickly, and their needs shift as they hit different developmental milestones. Recognizing when a routine requires adjustment is part of the parenting journey. Pay attention to signs that your baby's sleep patterns are changing or that they're ready for more extended periods of wakefulness. Celebrate these milestones, whether it's the first time they sleep through the night or their transition to solid foods. While sometimes challenging, these changes are opportunities for growth and bonding. Adapting to your baby's changing needs keeps you engaged and responsive, ensuring that routines remain beneficial and supportive for all of you.

As you settle into these new patterns, remember that routines are tools meant to serve you and your family, not rigid schedules to confine you. With patience and openness, you'll find a rhythm that works for your family, guiding you through the early days of parenthood.

Below is a general guide to normal newborn sleep, feeding, and wake patterns for the first six months of life.

Newborn Sleep, Feeding & Wake Patterns 0 – 6 Months

0-4 Weeks (Newborn Stage):
- **Total Sleep:** 16-18 hours per day
- **Day/Night Sleep:** Sleeps in short bursts (2-4 hours) throughout the day and night
- **Naps:** 4-6 per day
- **Wake Windows:** 45-60 minutes
- **Feeds:** Every 2-3 hours (8-12 feedings in 24 hours)
- **Key Notes:**
  - Sleep is highly fragmented due to hunger.
  - Day/night confusion is common.
  - Frequent diaper changes and burping are needed.

1-2 Months:
- **Total Sleep:** 14-17 hours per day
- **Day/Night Sleep:** Begins to consolidate longer night stretches (4-5 hours)
- **Naps:** 4-5 per day
- **Wake Windows:** 60-90 minutes
- **Feeds:** Every 2.5-3 hours (7-10 feedings in 24 hours)
- **Key Notes:**
  - Some babies start developing a more predictable wake/sleep cycle.
  - Longer night stretches (4-6 hours) may begin.
  - Gentle exposure to natural light can help regulate circadian rhythm.

2-3 Months:

- **Total Sleep:** 14-16 hours per day
- **Day/Night Sleep:** 5-7 hour stretches at night may develop.
- **Naps:** 4 per day
- **Wake Windows:** 75-90 minutes
- **Feeds:** Every 3-4 hours (6-8 feedings in 24 hours)
- **Key Notes:**
  - Babies begin showing signs of self-soothing.
  - Night sleep starts to consolidate into longer stretches.
  - There's more social interaction, cooing, and visual engagement.

3-4 Months (Sleep Regression Stage):

- **Total Sleep:** 14-16 hours per day
- **Day/Night Sleep:** Night stretches may shorten due to 4-month sleep regression.
- **Naps:** 3-4 per day
- **Wake Windows:** 90-120 minutes
- **Feeds:** Every 3-4 hours (5-7 feedings in 24 hours)
- **Key Notes:**
  - Sleep regression may occur due to brain development.
  - Baby is more aware of surroundings - can disrupt naps and night sleep.
  - Consistent bedtime routine helps.
  - May start rolling over—stop swaddling if baby is rolling.

4-5 Months:

- **Total Sleep:** 14-15 hours per day
- **Day/Night Sleep:** More solid 6–8-hour night stretches may develop.
- **Naps:** 3 per day
- **Wake Windows:** 1.5-2.5 hours
- **Feeds:** Every 3-4 hours (5-6 feedings in 24 hours)
- **Key Notes:**
  - Sleep training can begin if desired.
  - Teething may begin, causing brief night wakings.

5-6 Months:
- **Total Sleep:** 13-15 hours per day
- **Day/Night Sleep:** Nighttime sleep may reach 10-12 hours (with 1-2 feeds).
- **Naps:** 3 per day, eventually dropping to 2
- **Wake Windows:** 2-3 hours
- **Feeds:** Every 3-4 hours (5-6 feedings in 24 hours); may introduce solids per pediatrician advice
- **Key Notes:**
  - Baby may begin sleeping through the night with fewer night wakings.
  - A set sleep schedule with naps and a bedtime routine helps regulate sleep.
  - Baby is more mobile (rolling, scooting, early sitting up).
  - Solid foods should not replace milk/formula.

This guide serves as a general reference; always consult a pediatrician for concerns related to sleep, feeding, or developmental progress.

5

Building Team Chemistry – Connecting with Your Baby

The moment I first held my son, a nurse gently placed him in my arms and recommended I remove my shirt and hold him against my bare chest. This seemed an odd suggestion, but I followed her instructions. His tiny body was nestled against mine, his skin warm and soft, and I was blown away by how something so small could feel so monumental. This was more than just a physical connection; it was the beginning of a bond that would grow over a lifetime. As a new dad, you might be wondering how to forge such a connection with your newborn. One of the most profound ways to bond with your baby is through skin-to-skin contact. This simple yet powerful practice can set the stage for a lifetime of bonding and development.

Kickoff connection: Skin-to-skin contact

Skin-to-skin contact is a heartwarming experience and a major component in your baby's development. When you hold your baby against your chest, their tiny body adjusts to the world outside the womb. This contact helps regulate your baby's temperature and heart rate, keeping them warm and calm. According to the UNICEF UK Baby Friendly Initiative, this practice is essential for helping babies transition to life outside the womb. It can even stimulate digestion and enhance feeding interest, promoting breastfeeding success. When you hold your newborn close, you're not just providing comfort but actively supporting their physical development.

Engaging in skin-to-skin contact is most beneficial when initiated immediately after birth. The first hours are critical so doctors place babies directly on the mother's chest to help calm and relax the baby. Taking your turn of skin-to-skin contact promotes immediate bonding and sets the stage for your relationship. But don't limit this practice to just those early hours. Incorporating daily skin-to-skin routines can reinforce this bond. Whether after a bath or during a quiet moment, these sessions should become a regular part of your day.

The emotional connection created through skin-to-skin contact is profound. Holding your baby close builds trust and security, creating a safe space where they feel protected and loved. This act is mutually beneficial as it helps you develop a deeper emotional bond with your child. It's a reminder of the incredible responsibility and privilege of fatherhood. As your baby feels your warmth and hears your heartbeat, they're comforted by the familiarity of your presence. You, in turn, will experience a profound sense of connection and purpose. This shared experience will strengthen your relationship and lay the foundation for a strong bond that will grow over time.

Making skin-to-skin contact a habit requires intention and consistency. Getting caught up in the frenzy of work, running errands, diaper changes, feedings, and sleepless nights is easy, but carving out time for this simple practice is crucial. Set aside a few minutes each day to hold your baby against your chest. As you cradle your baby, take the time to breathe deeply, relax, and enjoy the connection you're building. These moments make all the challenges of fatherhood worthwhile.

Training time: Tummy time drills and their benefits

It's good for your little one to lie on their tummy, lifting their head to gaze around with curious eyes. This simple setup, known as tummy time, is more than just a cute sight—it's a vital part of their physical development. Tummy time helps strengthen your baby's neck and shoulder muscles, laying the foundation for rolling over, sitting up, and eventually crawling. It's basically their first gym session, where they begin to build the strength needed for all those exciting milestones ahead. Plus, it helps prevent flat spots on the head, a common issue when babies spend too much time on their backs. By encouraging these sessions, you're supporting their physical growth and promoting healthy motor skills that will benefit them as they grow.

Starting tummy time might seem daunting at first, but with a few simple steps, you can make it a safe and enjoyable experience for your baby. Choose a time when your baby is alert and content, perhaps after a nap or a diaper change. Place them on a soft, safe surface like a blanket on the floor. This provides a comfortable space for them to explore. Begin with short sessions, just a few minutes at a time, gradually increasing as they get stronger. Always stay close and supervise them, ready to offer encouragement and support. This ensures their safety and lets them know you're there, providing the comfort of your presence.

Try introducing interactive elements that capture your baby's attention to make tummy time more engaging. Place colorful toys just within reach, encouraging them to look and reach out. This makes the experience fun, stimulates their senses, and promotes hand-eye coordination. Get down on the floor with them, making it a joint activity. Talk to them, sing, or make funny faces. Your presence and interaction can transform tummy time from a chore into a delightful play session. These interactions help strengthen your bond and make the experience enjoyable for both of you.

Safety during tummy time is paramount, so always keep a watchful eye on your baby. Supervise them at all times, ensuring they're on a safe surface to prevent any accidents. Avoid having tummy time on elevated surfaces like beds or sofas, as these pose a risk of rolling off. Instead, opt for the floor or a play mat, where they can move freely without danger. Be attentive to their cues—if they seem tired or frustrated, take a break and try again later. These precautions ensure that tummy time remains a positive and beneficial part of your baby's daily routine.

Tummy Time Tracker

You may want to keep a tummy time tracker to monitor your baby's progress. Also, taking a short video with your phone is a good way to capture new tummy time milestones. This can be a rewarding way to see how your baby is developing, providing you with insights into their growth and achievements. Plus, it serves as a handy reminder to incorporate this practice regularly into your day.

Running early drills: Playing and interacting with your little teammate

As you gaze into your baby's eyes in those early days, a world of possibilities opens up. Play isn't just a way to pass time; it's a necessary part of your baby's development, laying the groundwork for cognitive skills and social awareness. Through play, your baby learns to interact with their environment, developing the ability to think, understand, and engage with others. It's a gentle introduction to the world around them, where every giggle and coo is a step towards understanding and connection. Playtime isn't just for fun—it's a building block for your baby's future learning and growth.

Consider starting with simple, age-appropriate activities that create opportunities for bonding. Peek-a-boo is a classic, and for good reason. The simple act of covering your face and then revealing it with a smile can elicit pure joy from your little one. This game helps your baby start to understand the concept that things continue to exist even when they're out of sight. Gentle tickling, too, can bring smiles and laughter, cultivating a sense of trust and safety. Exploring textures is another engaging activity; try offering different toys with various feels, like soft fabric or bumpy rubber. These textures stimulate your baby's senses, encouraging them to explore the world around them with their tiny hands.

Facial expressions and vocalizations play a significant role in these interactions. Making eye contact and smiling at your baby is a simple yet powerful way to convey love and affection. Your facial expressions are signals that communicate emotions and reactions your baby can mimic and learn from. Similarly, your voice is an instrument of connection. Mimicking your baby's sounds encourages cooing and babbling and lays the foundation for language development. Your voice is their first introduction to the nuances of communication, helping them understand tone, pitch, and rhythm. These interactions are fun and they're vital for teaching your baby how to express themselves.

As a dad, you can be creative, inventing games and activities that cater to your baby's interests. It's quite well known that dads always get to be the fun parent, so take advantage of that role! Notice what captures their attention—is it a particular toy, a funny noise, or a silly face? Use these cues to create personalized play experiences. Maybe your baby loves it when you make animal sounds or blow fart noises on their belly. These moments are opportunities for innovation, allowing you to tailor playtime to your baby's preferences. Don't be afraid to try new things and see what makes them light up – just be sure to keep it safe.

Remember, play is a shared adventure, a chance to explore and learn together. It's about being present and engaged, creating a safe space where your baby feels free to express themselves. Each playful moment is a step towards building a strong, loving bond with your baby, a foundation to support them as they grow and discover the world.

Building the foundation: Reading and singing with your baby early

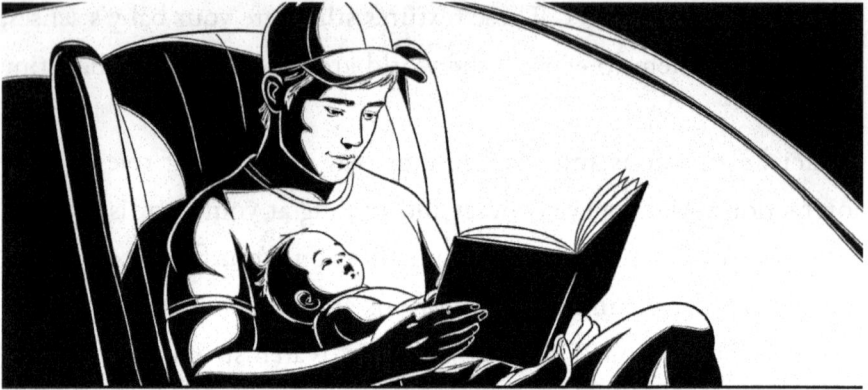

You're sitting in the nursery, a soft glow from the nightlight casting gentle shadows on the wall. Your baby is cradled in your arms, eyes wide with wonder as you open a picture book and begin to read. Though perhaps not fully understood, each word wraps them in the warmth of your voice. Reading and singing to your baby might seem simple, but it is foundational for language development and emotional bonding. When you read stories, you introduce a world of vocabulary, every word is a key drill that powers their imagination and strengthens their growing mind. Stories become a gateway to language, exposing them to new sounds and patterns that aid in cognitive growth. And let's not forget the soothing power of a gentle lullaby. Singing creates a calming routine that can ease your baby into a restful sleep, turning those nightly rituals into cherished moments of connection. Plus, your baby won't judge if you don't have a perfect singing voice—they'll just appreciate the comfort of your presence.

Incorporating reading and singing into daily life doesn't have to be a difficult task—it can fit naturally into the rhythm of your day. Establish a bedtime story ritual, a peaceful end to the day that signals it's time to wind down. Take nightly turns with your partner, so you are actively involved. Choose books with colorful graphics and simple text that capture their attention. The familiarity of a favorite story can bring comfort, making bedtime something they look forward to. Be prepared to read the same story over and over—little ones love repetition! But don't stop there. Sing to your baby during diaper changes or bath time. Your familiar and reassuring voice can transform these routine tasks into opportunities for bonding. The songs don't have to be complex; even a simple, repetitive tune can work wonders. These melodies become a soundtrack to their daily life, creating an auditory connection that strengthens your relationship.

Your voice is your greatest tool when it comes to reading and singing. Using varied tones and expressions can captivate your baby's attention and make the experience more engaging. Think of your voice as an instrument capable of conveying different emotions. A gentle whisper can calm, while an animated tone can excite. As you read, emphasize specific words, changing your pitch or speed to keep them engaged. When singing, play with volume and tempo, experimenting to see what your baby responds to. These changes in voice help them discern different sounds, building early language skills and emotional recognition.

Repetition and consistency are key to making these interactions meaningful. Babies thrive on routine, and repeatedly hearing the same stories or songs helps build familiarity and comfort. While it might feel monotonous to you, it's laying the groundwork for their understanding. Over time, they begin to anticipate the next page in a story or the chorus of a song, delighting in the predictability and security it brings. So, make it a habit. Dedicate a few minutes daily to these activities, creating a space for connection and learning. Through reading and singing, you're doing more than communicating; you're building a bridge of love and understanding that will support their growth and development.

Reading the play: Recognizing and responding to your baby's signals

You're rocking your baby gently, and they begin to squirm, making little rooting motions with their mouth. All moms know this cue quite well. This is one of the many cues your baby will give you—a subtle sign that they might be hungry. Recognizing these cues is like learning a new language, one that helps you understand your baby's needs before they resort to crying. Hunger cues can range from rooting and sucking motions to fussing or even smacking their lips. On the other hand, when your baby starts yawning or rubbing their eyes, they're likely letting you know it's time for some shut-eye. These signals are your baby's way of communicating and being attuned to them can make a world of difference.

Responding to these cues promptly is crucial for building trust and security. When your baby realizes their needs are met swiftly, they begin to understand that they're in a safe, nurturing environment. Picking up your baby when they cry isn't just about quieting them down; it's about reinforcing their sense of security. Each time you respond, you teach them that their world is a predictable, safe place where their needs are acknowledged and met. This trust builds the foundation of a strong bond that grows deeper with every interaction. It's an investment in their emotional well-being, promoting a sense of safety and love.

Decoding these cues might seem challenging to new dads at first, but with a bit of observation, patterns begin to emerge. Start by watching your baby closely throughout the day. Take note of when they show hunger cues and how they progress to crying if not addressed. Similarly, observe their sleep cues and how they transition from being alert to drowsy. Moms are often really good at recognizing cues so consulting with your wife or partner is invaluable in this process. This collaboration enhances your ability to interpret cues and strengthens your parenting partnership.

Overtime strategy: Understanding your baby's needs in the fourth quarter

Imagine entering a new world where everything is suddenly bright, loud, and unfamiliar. This is the fourth trimester for your newborn—a pivotal period where they adjust to life outside the womb. It's a time when your baby still craves the warmth and comfort they knew before birth. They're learning to regulate their body temperature, breathing, and even digestion, all tasks that were once effortlessly handled within the womb. This transition can affect their behavior, leading to fussiness or frequent waking as they adapt to their new environment. Your role during this time is to create a nurturing atmosphere that eases this shift and provides the comfort and security they need to feel safe.

Creating a nurturing environment is key to supporting your baby through the fourth trimester. Think of it as recreating the womb's warmth and security in your home. Snuggly swaddling your baby can provide that sense of security they miss, mimicking the gentle pressure they felt before birth. This technique helps soothe them, reducing startle reflexes that might wake them from sleep. The gentle motion of rocking or using a baby carrier can also work wonders in calming your little one. This rhythmic movement is reminiscent of the gentle swaying they experienced while nestled inside the womb. These small, steady motions can become integral to soothing them and making them feel secure. Another useful tool is white noise, which can drown out household sounds and replicate the whooshing noise they listened to in utero. These soothing sounds can calm your baby, helping them settle more quickly. Your home becomes a sanctuary, a place where your baby can unwind and adjust gradually to the unfamiliar world around them.

It's normal for you to feel frustrated or exhausted but remember that your baby is navigating an entirely new world. Patience, attentiveness, empathy, and understanding are your greatest allies during these early months. Babies are constantly changing, and their cues often evolve as they grow. What worked yesterday might not work today, so you'll need to be adaptable. It's a learning process that requires an open mind. Remember, there's no one-size-fits-all approach to parenting. Be patient with yourself as you practice this new language, knowing that each attempt brings you closer to understanding your baby. The more attentive you are, the more you'll learn about what makes your little one tick. Hold your baby close, offering comfort and reassurance as they explore this unfamiliar environment. Compassion is key, not just towards your baby, but also towards yourself and your wife or partner. You're all learning together, figuring out what works best for your family. There will be good days and challenging ones, but with each hurdle, you'll gain confidence as a parent.

These early weeks are a time of adjustment for everyone. As you wrap up this chapter on understanding your baby's immediate needs, consider how these foundational practices—creating a nurturing environment, addressing their needs with patience, and practicing empathy—set the stage for the parenting journey ahead. The next chapter will continue to build on these principles, exploring how to care for your newborn with love and attentiveness.

6

Leveling Up Your Parenting Skills and Newborn Care

B ecoming a new dad is like stepping onto the court for the championship game—thrilling, a little intimidating, and packed with unexpected plays. And if there's one ride you'll find yourself on more often than any other, it's the diaper duty express. It involves mastering a skill that will become second nature in no time. You might not win any awards for it, but becoming a pro at diaper changes is a badge of honor in the world of parenting. Let's dive into the nitty-gritty of diaper duty and turn this essential task into a bonding moment with your baby.

Crushing diaper duty: Pro tips for the win

When choosing the correct diaper, the options can be overwhelming. The main decision boils down to cloth versus disposable. However, you don't have to choose one type over the other. Cloth diapers are eco-friendly and cost-effective over time, while disposables offer convenience and ease, especially when you're on the go. Most families today choose disposable diapers. If you opt for disposables, there are popular brands like Pampers, Huggies, and Luvs. However, according to a review by Wirecutter, other brands, such as Parent's Choice and Up & Up, provide excellent performance at a budget-friendly price. Whichever you choose, the key is finding the right fit. Diapers should be snug but not tight, hugging comfortably around the waist and legs to prevent leaks. Size matters, too; as your baby grows, the diaper size will need to adjust accordingly.

Hygiene is fundamental in diaper duty. Each change should include a thorough cleaning to prevent irritation and diaper rash. Use gentle wipes or a damp washcloth to clean the baby's skin, ensuring all areas are dry before putting on a new diaper. Preventing diaper rash involves keeping the skin dry and applying a thin layer of protective cream if needed. Look for creams with zinc oxide, as they create a barrier against moisture. Some good examples are Desitin, Boudreaux's Butt Paste, and A+D Diaper Rash Cream. Regular checks and changes are the best defense against irritation, so aim to change the diaper every two to three hours or whenever it's soiled.

Below is a simple guide that walks you through the steps of changing a baby's diaper.

***

Diaper Duty Guide:

Follow these steps to safely and comfortably change your baby's diaper.

1. Gather Your Supplies

- Before you begin, make sure you have everything you need within arm's reach.
- Clean diaper, wipes, diaper cream, changing pad or soft surface, plastic bag for disposal.
- Change of clothes for baby if anything has leaked through the soiled diaper.

2. Position the Baby

- Gently lay the baby down on their back on a safe, clean surface (changing pad).
- Always keep one hand on the baby to prevent them from rolling off.

3. Remove the Dirty Diaper

- Unfasten the tabs of the dirty diaper.
- Gently lift the baby's legs by the ankles and pull the dirty diaper away from under them.
- Use the front part of the dirty diaper to wipe away any excess mess, folding it over itself.

4. Clean the Baby

- Use baby wipes to clean the baby thoroughly.
- Always wipe from front to back to prevent infection.
- Make sure to clean all the folds and creases and allow skin to dry completely.

5. Apply Diaper Cream (if needed)

- If the baby has a rash or if you want to prevent one, apply a thin layer of diaper cream as per the instructions on the product.

6. Place the New Diaper

- Slide a fresh diaper under the baby, ensuring the back is higher than the front.
- Position the tabs at the baby's waist.
- Bring the front of the diaper up between the baby's legs.

7. Secure the Diaper

- Secure the tabs to the front of the diaper, ensuring a snug fit but not too tight.
- Check to ensure the leg openings are secure to prevent leaks.

8. Dispose of the Dirty Diaper

- Roll up the dirty diaper and secure it with the tabs.
- Place it in a plastic bag and seal it before disposing of it in the trash.
- Wash your hands thoroughly.

Common challenges, like diaper rash, can be a source of frustration. If irritation occurs, applying a protective cream can soothe the skin. Give the baby some diaper-free time—tummy time is a good opportunity—to let their skin breathe. If the rash persists, consult your pediatrician for advice as an anti-fungal cream may be needed. Staying positive during diaper changes turns this routine task into a moment of connection. Sing or talk to your baby, narrate your actions, or tell a silly story. Play music or offer a small toy for distraction. These interactions entertain your little one and strengthen your bond, turning a simple diaper change into a cherished moment.

Create a checklist to keep by the changing station. Include baby items like clean diapers, wipes, cream, and a changing pad. Add reminders to check for leaks and ensure supplies are restocked regularly. This checklist can be a handy reference, making diaper duty more efficient and stress-free. Below is a simple Changing Station Checklist example.

Simple Diaper Duty Checklist for Baby's Changing Station:

1. Diapering Essentials:

- **Diapers**: Keep a stack of the right size and type for your baby.
- **Wipes**: Choose fragrance-free or sensitive-skin wipes if preferred.
- **Diaper Cream/Ointment**: For preventing and treating rashes.
- **Changing Pad**: A wipeable surface or a pad with removable covers.

2. Extras:

- **Disposable Bags or Diaper Pail**: For quick and odor-free disposal.
- **Hand Sanitizer**: In case you can't wash your hands immediately.
- **Burp Cloth or Cloth Wipes**: Helpful for cleanup.
- **Change of Clothes**: In case of accidents.

3. Safety First:

- **Always Keep One Hand on Baby**: Never leave baby unattended.
- **Strap or Guardrails (if available)**: Use them for added security.

4. Clean-Up Routine:

- **Wipe Down Changing Surface:** After each use.
- **Restock Supplies:** Check diaper and wipe levels daily.
- **Wash Hands Thoroughly**: To prevent spreading germs.

5. Optional Items:

- **Distraction Toys:** Small toys or rattles to keep baby occupied.
- **Night Light**: Useful for late-night changes.

Keep these items within arm's reach and ensure the area is always tidy to make diaper changes quick, safe, and stress-free.

Swaddling like a pro

Swaddling might seem like an ancient art, but its benefits for a newborn are very modern and real. Imagine being wrapped in a warm, gentle hug—that's what swaddling offers your baby. It recreates the cozy security of the womb, helping your little one feel calm and secure, which can lead to better sleep and reduced fussiness. Babies have a startle reflex that can wake them up, but swaddling keeps their arms snug, preventing this reflex from interrupting their rest. The key is to swaddle correctly, ensuring comfort without restricting movement or causing safety issues.

***

How to Swaddle a Baby

Follow these steps to safely and comfortably swaddle your baby.

1. Choose the Right Swaddle Blanket

- The ideal size is 42x42 inches, no larger than 47x47 inches.
- Choose a soft, thin, breathable material like cotton.
- Lay the blanket on a flat surface in a diamond shape and fold the top corner down.

2. Position the Baby

- Place your baby face up on the blanket.
- Ensure their neck aligns with the folded edge.

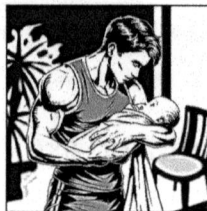

3. Position Their Arms

- Gently place their arms by their sides for comfort and safety.

4. Wrap the Right Side

- Pull the right side of the blanket across the baby's body diagonally.
- Tuck it snugly under the opposite side.

5. Fold Up the Bottom Corner

- Bring the bottom corner over the baby's feet.
- Ensure there is enough room for hip and leg movement to prevent hip dysplasia.

6. Secure with the Left Side

- Wrap the left side diagonally over and under the baby.
- Make sure the swaddle is snug but not too tight, allowing for breathing and movement.

Swaddling can help comfort your baby and promote better sleep. Always monitor your baby to ensure they remain safely swaddled and comfortable.

Here are some additional pro tips for swaddling your little teammate:

- Always swaddle your baby on their back to promote safe sleep.

- Swaddle with their arms positioned down and to their sides.

- Swaddling helps relax babies and protect them from overheating, injuries, and SIDS during the early months after birth.

If traditional swaddling feels intimidating, some alternatives might suit your baby better. Swaddle wraps or sleep sacks can simplify the process. These products often come with Velcro or zippers, making them easy to use. They provide the same sense of security while ensuring the swaddle stays intact, even for the wiggliest babies. Some sleep sacks also allow for arms to be left out, which can be helpful if your baby prefers more freedom. Experiment with different methods to see what works best for your little one, as every baby has their own preferences.

Safety is paramount when it comes to swaddling. A snug fit is essential, but the swaddle should never be so tight that it restricts breathing or movement. A good rule of thumb is to ensure you can fit two fingers between the swaddle and your baby's chest. Overheating is another concern, so always use lightweight materials and dress your baby in minimal clothing underneath the swaddle. Monitor room temperature and adjust as needed to keep your baby comfortable. Swaddling should stop when your baby shows signs of rolling over, as this increases the risk of suffocation. This is typically between two and four months of age. At this stage, transitioning to a sleep sack that allows for unrestricted arm movement is a safe alternative.

Bathtime strategy: Keeping it safe and comfortable

Most authorities recommend simply sponge bathing your baby until their umbilical cord has dried and fallen off to prevent infection. Others feel it's fine to bath your newborn provided you dry the cord area afterwards. Whatever you decide, bathtime with your little one can be an enjoyable experience filled with giggles and splashes. However, you must set up a safe and soothing environment before the fun begins. Start by designating a specific bathing area, whether in the bathroom or in the kitchen. Ensure all supplies are within arm's reach: a baby bathtub, mild baby soap, a soft washcloth, and a few towels. Safety is paramount, so always test the water temperature before placing your baby in the tub. Aim for about 100°F, which is warm enough to be comfortable but not too hot. Opt for gentle, fragrance-free baby products to avoid irritating your newborn's sensitive skin.

Once everything's set, it's time to confidently bathe your baby. Support their head and neck with one hand as you gently lower them into the water, using your other hand to secure their little body. Begin by washing their face with a damp washcloth, avoiding soap near the eyes. Use mild baby soap for the rest of their body, gently lathering and rinsing as you go. Be sure to clean their skin folds, where milk and sweat can accumulate. After a thorough wash, carefully lift your baby out of the bath and wrap them snugly in a warm towel. Pat them dry, especially in the creases, to prevent irritation. A light application of baby lotion can help keep their skin soft and moisturized.

Bath time can present a few challenges that might catch you off guard. Babies are naturally slippery when wet, so maintaining a secure grip is vital. Hold them securely with one hand supporting their head and shoulders while washing with the other, and never leave them unattended in the water. Introducing your baby to water can be tricky; some love it, while others need time to adjust. It helps if the room is warm. Gradually ease them into the experience by pouring a small amount of water over their body before fully immersing them. It's also common for babies to urinate or have a bowel movement during bath time. If this happens, calmly remove them from the water, clean them up, and refresh the bath.

Transform bath time into a bonding session by creating a relaxing atmosphere. Introduce soft bath toys to engage your baby and make the experience enjoyable. Singing or talking to them during the bath can soothe their nerves and promote a sense of security. Dimming the lights or playing gentle music adds to the calming ambiance, turning what could be a routine task into quality time with your little champ. This is not just about cleanliness; it's a chance to connect and share in the simple joy of being together.

Newborn hygiene: Covering the fundamentals

As you handle the ups and downs of caring for a newborn, maintaining good hygiene is critical to keeping your baby healthy and happy.

Umbilical Cord

Pay special attention to the umbilical cord area, which needs to remain clean and dry until it naturally falls off, typically within the first few weeks. Use a damp cotton ball or swab to gently clean around the base, being careful not to tug at it. Avoid submerging your baby in water until the cord has completely healed to prevent any risk of infection.

Nail Care

Nail care is another important aspect of newborn hygiene, as those tiny nails can be surprisingly sharp. Use a pair of baby nail clippers or a file to keep them trimmed and smooth. It's often easiest to do this when your baby is asleep and less likely to squirm around. Be patient and take your time—accidents happen, and it's all part of the learning curve.

Stuffy Noses

For stuffy noses, a nasal aspirator or bulb syringe can help clear congestion. Squeeze the bulb before gently inserting it into the nostril, then release it to draw out mucus. Fair warning: don't get overwhelmed if your baby cries and fusses when suctioning out their little nose. All babies hate it.

However, this can be especially helpful during colds or when your baby has trouble breathing comfortably.

Cradle Cap

Cradle cap is when crusty white or yellow scales form on the baby's head. It's probably caused by excessive oil production around the hair follicles but it's harmless. Preventing cradle cap involves regularly washing your baby's scalp with mild shampoo and gently brushing the hair to remove any flakes. It's a common condition that usually clears up on its own, but these steps can help manage it.

Baby Acne

Baby acne might appear as tiny red or white bumps on your baby's face. It's typically harmless and doesn't require treatment beyond regular gentle cleansing with water. Never squeeze the little spots!

Bottle & Pacifier Sanitization

Hygiene also includes bottle and pacifier sanitization, something very important to prevent tummy upsets. Wash the bottles in hot soapy water then boil them after every feeding. Alternatively, put them in the dishwasher. Pacifiers should also be boiled regularly, especially if they fall on the floor or come into contact with unwashed surfaces. You can also use a sterilizer for these items to ensure they're free from germs.

Perfect plays to calm a fussy baby

Being faced with a fussy baby can feel like you've struck out. You're sleep-deprived, and your little one won't stop crying. However, understanding the root causes of their fussiness is the first step in finding a solution. More often than not, hunger or discomfort tops the list. Babies have small stomachs, so they get hungry frequently. A missed feeding or a diaper that's a little too snug can lead to tears. Then there's gas or reflux—digestive issues that can make your baby very uncomfortable. A gentle tummy massage or holding them upright after feedings can help alleviate some of that discomfort. Overstimulation is another culprit. Babies are learning to process the world around them, and when there's too much happening, they can become overwhelmed. Sometimes, they're simply tired, and some quiet time is all they need. Recognizing these signs can help you address their needs effectively.

Once you've identified the possible reason for their distress, introducing calming techniques can work wonders. Gentle rocking or bouncing is often the go-to solution. It mimics the soothing motion of the womb and can help lull your baby back to calmness. If you have a rocking chair or glider, now's the time to make it your best friend. Alternatively, carrying your baby in a sling while walking can also soothe them. The gentle sway and your closeness can be incredibly comforting. A pacifier can also serve as a source of comfort. It satisfies the natural sucking reflex and can often soothe a baby who's not necessarily hungry but needs to self-soothe. Experiment with these techniques to see what your baby responds to best.

The atmosphere in your home also determines how easily your baby can be soothed. A change in surroundings can make all the difference. Dimming the lights or switching on lamps instead of bright overhead lights can reduce stimulation, creating a calming atmosphere that signals it's time to relax. Soft, calming music or white noise can also be helpful. The rhythmic sounds can distract and soothe, helping your baby settle down. You might want to create a playlist of gentle tunes or invest in a white noise machine. Sometimes, simply changing rooms or stepping outside for a moment can offer a fresh perspective for you and the baby. These easy environmental adjustments can turn a chaotic moment into a peaceful one.

As mentioned in earlier chapters, patience, persistence, and flexibility are your best allies. It's easy to feel frustrated when nothing seems to work, but remember that each baby is unique. What works for one may not work for another, and finding the right combination of techniques can take time. Keep trying different strategies with a calm demeanor. Your baby picks up on your energy, so staying relaxed can help them feel more secure. Celebrate the small victories, even if they're just a few minutes of quiet. Each moment of calm is a step toward understanding your baby better. You're learning together, and with patience, you'll find the rhythm that works for you both.

Running offense during growth spurts and cluster feedings

You've just started getting the hang of life with a newborn when, suddenly, your little one becomes a tiny eating machine. Worst yet, Mom is out running errands, you have a limited supply of expressed breastmilk or prepared formula, and you're home alone watching the baby. Welcome to the world of growth spurts! During these times, babies often experience a significant increase in appetite. You might wonder if you've somehow brought home a very small teenager, given how frequently they want to feed. This is perfectly normal. Growth spurts often coincide with developmental milestones and require more energy, hence the increased hunger. These spurts typically occur at about three weeks, six weeks, three months, and six months of age, but these are averages. Every baby is unique, and yours might not follow this exact schedule.

Enter cluster feeding, a phenomenon that often accompanies growth spurts and can leave you feeling like you're on a constant loop of feeding, burping, and changing. Cluster feeding involves your baby wanting to feed more frequently over a short period. It's their way of ensuring they get enough nutrition to fuel their rapid growth. You'll recognize it when your baby demands feedings every hour or two, especially during the evening. It can be exhausting, but responding to their hunger cues and feeding on demand is essential.

Managing these intense periods without losing your sanity requires a bit of strategy. Flexibility with feeding schedules is key. Forget the clock and focus on your baby's cues. If they're hungry, feed them—simple as that. It might mean shorter intervals between feeds, but this is temporary. Ensuring both parents get adequate rest is crucial during this time. Tag team the duties when possible, allowing each parent to recharge. Even short power naps can make a big difference in your energy levels. Consider sharing night feeds if you're bottle-feeding, or find other ways to support each other through these demanding days.

In addition to their voracious appetite, you might notice changes in sleep patterns during growth spurts. Your baby may sleep more than usual as their body works hard to grow and develop. Alternatively, some babies become fussier and have a tougher time settling down. This can be challenging for parents, but understanding that these behaviors are linked to growth can help ease your concerns. It's a time when patience becomes your best friend as you handle these phases of rapid development. Remember, the extra feeding and sleep disturbances are temporary and essential for your baby's development.

The good news is that growth spurts are temporary. They come in waves, and once they pass, your baby will often settle back into a more predictable routine. It's a natural part of their development, ensuring they grow strong and healthy. As challenging as these times can be, they're also a testament to your baby's progress. Embrace the changes, knowing that they're signs of growth and development. Just when you think you've reached your wit's end, you'll find a new rhythm. Your baby will emerge from these spurts with new skills and abilities, ready to explore the world in new ways. As you move forward, remember that each phase, no matter how taxing, is a stepping stone in your baby's journey to becoming who they're meant to be. With growth spurts behind us, it's time to explore the world of sleep training in the next chapter.

Step Up & Make an Impact—Leave a Review

"The impact you make today can change someone's life tomorrow." – **Unknown**

When you were looking for guidance, what brought you here to *Dad Rookie*? Was it a recommendation from a fellow dad-to-be or maybe a standout review? The truth is, most people choose books based on what others say about them. Your words might be the reason another first-time dad picks up *Dad Rookie* and walks into fatherhood with confidence instead of confusion and doubt.

If you are enjoying *Dad Rookie* so far and feel it has helped you in any way, I'd be incredibly grateful if you'd take a moment to leave a quick review. It doesn't have to be long—just a few words on what you have liked and found helpful so far.

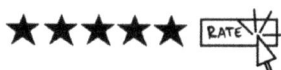

★★★★★ RATE

Simply scan the QR code below to leave a review and share your thoughts:

You've already taken the first step in being a great dad by investing in yourself. Now, you have the chance to help another rookie do the same. Thank you for being a part of the *Dad Rookie* team. You're making a big impact!

Your teammate in fatherhood, Lane Carter

7

Bedtime Game Plan – Mastering Newborn Sleep Strategies

Y ou're standing over the crib trying to keep your eyes open, the moonlight is casting soft shadows across the room, and you wonder if your little guy will ever sleep for more than a few hours. You're not alone in this nocturnal adventure. Many new dads struggle with newborn sleep patterns, trying to decipher why their little one wakes so frequently or why day and night seem interchangeable to them. Understanding these sleep patterns is like unraveling a mystery. Still, it's a puzzle worth solving for your and your partner's sanity.

Breaking it down: Understanding sleep patterns

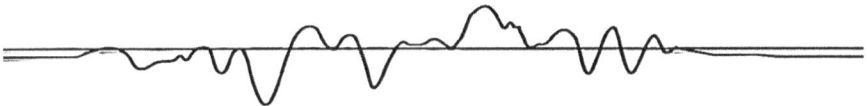

In the early weeks, newborn sleep is erratic. You might notice your baby's sleep is characterized by short cycles and frequent awakenings. These waking moments are often dictated by their need for feeding or diaper changing, and your newborn may sleep anywhere from 12 to 16 hours within 24 hours, broken into multiple short naps. Unlike adults, newborns have immature circadian rhythms, which means they can't distinguish between day and night. You might find that your baby sleeps for longer periods during the day and has shorter, more frequent naps at night. You might find yourself wide awake at 2 a.m., soothing a wide-eyed infant who believes it's time to party. It's not that your baby is being difficult; their internal clock simply hasn't adjusted to the norms we live by. This is perfectly normal and part of their learning process. As your baby grows, these sleep durations will gradually lengthen, and they'll start consolidating their sleep into longer stretches.

As you adapt to your new dad role, it's important to remember that these irregular sleep-wake patterns are entirely normal. A newborn's sleep cycle includes active and quiet sleep phases, with active sleep being a time of movement and noise and quiet sleep being more restful. These cycles can last anywhere from 20 to 50 minutes. During these active sleep phases, you'll observe your baby's eyes moving under their eyelids, little limbs twitching, and perhaps even small sounds escaping their lips. This is all part of their development, and while it may seem disruptive, it's how they process and respond to the world around them.

Bedtime warm-ups: Getting ready for the big wind-down

In the fast-paced hustle of being a new dad, establishing a sleep routine can feel like finding a lighthouse in a storm. It's not just about getting your baby to sleep—it's about creating a rhythm that calms the entire household. Routine gives your baby a sense of security and predictability, something essential in their rapidly changing world. When you consistently set a regular bedtime and wake-up time, you're teaching your baby what to expect, which can help them feel more secure and relaxed. Predictability is calming, like a steady game plan that reassures your baby, "You're safe. We've got this."

The magic of a sleep routine lies in its consistency. Consistency helps regulate your baby's internal clock, aligning it more closely with the natural day-night cycle. This doesn't happen overnight, but with regular cues, such as dimming the lights, a warm bath, or a lullaby, your baby begins to associate these activities with sleep. Over time, these cues help signal to your baby that it's time to wind down, making the transition to sleep smoother. Imagine how comforting it is for your baby to know that after a bath and a story, it's time to snuggle down and drift off. It turns bedtime into a peaceful process rather than a nightly battle.

For your new family, a well-established routine offers the benefit of predictability. You can plan your evenings knowing roughly when your baby will be asleep. This time becomes a precious window for you to relax, connect with each other, or simply enjoy a moment of quiet. The predictability of a routine can help reduce the stress and chaos that often accompany those early weeks of parenting. It sets the stage for a calmer, more organized life where chaos doesn't reign supreme. Plus, once your baby's routine is set, you'll likely find that they sleep better and wake up happier, ready to explore the world with curious eyes.

Creating this routine requires trial and error. Start by observing your baby's natural rhythms and preferences. Do they seem more relaxed after a bath? Do they enjoy a story before sleep? Use these observations to create a routine that suits your baby's disposition. You might find that a gentle massage with baby lotion helps calm them down, or perhaps they respond well to a particular lullaby. Whatever it is, incorporate these elements consistently, allowing your baby to create associations between these activities and sleep.

Consistency doesn't mean rigidity. Life with a newborn is unpredictable, and some nights will inevitably deviate from the plan. That's okay. The aim is to create a routine that is flexible enough to adapt to your baby's changing needs. Some nights require more soothing, while others might unfold seamlessly. The key is to maintain the core elements of your routine, even if the timing shifts. This flexibility is necessary for keeping your sanity as a parent, helping you roll with the punches while still providing your baby with the comfort of familiar rituals.

There will be nights when your baby resists sleep despite your best efforts. This doesn't mean you're doing anything wrong; it's simply part of the process. Stick with it, and over time, you'll likely notice these disruptions become less frequent. Remember, the goal isn't to achieve perfection but to create an environment where your baby feels safe and loved. In these routine moments, you're not just preparing your baby for sleep—you're also laying the foundation for trust and security.

Conquering sleep challenges: A winning strategy for dads

Day/Night Confusion

Traversing the world of newborn sleep can feel like tiptoeing through a minefield. One moment, your little one is sleeping soundly, and the next, they're wide awake, seemingly ready to conquer the world. Day/night confusion is one of the first hurdles you'll likely encounter. Your baby can seem like a tiny night owl who plays under the stars and naps throughout the day. This confusion stems from the fact that your baby's internal clock hasn't entirely adjusted to our 24-hour cycle. This can lead to unpredictable sleeping hours, with your baby often being more unsettled during the late afternoon and evening. It may feel like as soon as you get them settled, they're awake again, ready for the next feed or change. To help them differentiate, create clear distinctions between day and night. During the day, keep the environment lively and bright. Engage your baby with activities and allow natural light to fill the room. This exposure will help them learn that daytime is for activity. In contrast, keep nighttime feedings quiet and low-stimulation. Use dim lighting, avoid play, and speak softly.

These cues signal your baby that it's time to sleep, not engage. Over time, usually by around three months, your baby will start to adjust, and their sleep patterns will begin to stabilize. These strategies, though simple, can transform your nights into something more restful and less chaotic, setting the stage for healthy sleep habits that will serve them well beyond these early months.

Short Sleep Cycles

Short sleep cycles can also throw a wrench into your plans. Newborns naturally have these short cycles, leading to frequent waking. It's as if they've come pre-installed with a snooze button that gets hit every 45 minutes. The trick here is to respond quickly and calmly when they wake, offering comfort without unnecessary stimulation. Keeping things low-key helps prevent overstimulation, which can make it harder for them to drift back to sleep. Think of it as quietly resetting the scene each time they stir, setting the stage for them to fall back into slumber without much fuss.

Cluster Feeding

As we discussed in Chapter 6, cluster feeding is another common challenge that affects newborn sleep patterns, especially in the evenings. Cluster feedings are your baby's way of stocking up for the night ahead. While it can be exhausting, this pattern is often temporary. During these periods, your baby is likely going through a growth spurt, needing more nourishment to fuel their rapid development. Remember to forget the clock and focus on your baby's cues. If they're hungry, feed them. Also, tag team the duties when possible, allowing each parent to recharge and refresh. Try sharing night feeds if you're bottle-feeding, or find other ways to support each other through the first demanding months.

Frequent Night Wakings

Frequent night waking is part and parcel of life with a newborn. While it might feel relentless, it's completely normal. Your baby's need for feeding or comfort is a natural part of their development. Responding swiftly can prevent them from fully waking and help you both get back to sleep quicker. The key is to keep these interactions brief and soothing, minimizing disruptions to their sleep cycle.

Overtiredness/Overstimulation

Recognizing signs of overtiredness is important. An overtired baby can become fussy and harder to settle, much like an exhausted adult who can't seem to unwind. Look for cues like rubbing eyes, fussiness, or disengagement. Catching these signs early on allows you to take them to a quiet space and put them down for a nap before they become too overstimulated. Your baby is a sponge, soaking up all the sights, sounds, and interactions around them. When there's too much going on, that sponge overflows, leading to a frazzled baby who struggles to settle. Removing them to a calm, soothing environment can help prevent this, providing a serene backdrop for sleep.

The Moro Reflex

The startle reflex, or Moro reflex, is another quirk of newborn sleep. It's as if your baby suddenly feels like they're falling, leading to flailing arms and disrupted sleep. Swaddling can help contain these movements, offering the security they need to stay asleep. It's like providing a gentle hug that keeps them from startling themselves awake.

Feeding Dependency

Feeding to sleep is a common habit that can lead to dependency. While wanting to soothe your baby with a feed is natural, it's important to gradually encourage self-soothing. This means finding other ways to settle your baby to sleep, like gentle rocking or a soft lullaby, so they don't rely solely on feeding to drift off.

Colic

Colic or tummy discomfort can also disrupt sleep. A fussy, colicky baby can seem inconsolable, but there are ways to ease their discomfort. Try gentle rocking, burping, or a soothing massage to help alleviate their distress. Sometimes a warm bath helps. Each baby is unique, so finding the perfect combination that works for your little one might take some trial and error.

Sleep Strategies

Sudden Unexplained Infant Deaths (SUIDs) refer to the sudden and unexplained death of an infant, often during sleep, and can encompass conditions like Sudden Infant Death Syndrome (SIDS). While the exact cause remains unknown, certain practices can significantly reduce the risk. One of the most reassuring newborn sleep tools at your disposal is the concept of safe sleep practices. The "ABCs" of safe sleep provide a straightforward guide: babies should sleep **A**lone, on their **B**ack, in a **C**rib or bassinet. This setup minimizes risks associated with SUIDs and offers peace of mind during those early months. Avoid co-sleeping or laying your baby on soft surfaces like couches or adult beds. These environments can pose suffocation hazards. Instead, use a firm mattress with a tightly fitted sheet, keeping the crib free from pillows, blankets, and stuffed animals. A swaddle or sleep sack can be a comforting addition, providing warmth and security without the risk of loose bedding.

To assist with daytime napping, the Eat-Play-Sleep Cycle offers a helpful strategy for organizing your baby's day. The cycle involves three simple steps: feed, play, and sleep. After your baby wakes, start by feeding them. This ensures they're full and content, ready to engage with their environment. Next, incorporate a little playtime. This doesn't need to be elaborate—a gentle interaction like singing or showing them a colorful object can work wonders. Finally, as you notice signs of tiredness, like yawning or rubbing eyes, it's time to put them down for a nap. This pattern helps separate feeding from sleeping, preventing your baby from associating feeding with falling asleep. Over time, this separation can encourage more sustainable sleep habits, making it easier for your baby to settle without needing to eat.

Encouraging self-soothing is way to promote longer sleep stretches. This doesn't mean leaving your baby to cry but instead allowing them to fall asleep on their own. Try placing them in their crib when they're drowsy but still awake. This helps them associate the crib with sleep and learn to settle themselves. Over time, this approach can reduce the need for your intervention, helping them develop independent sleep skills. It's a gradual process, but it lays a solid foundation for future sleep success.

Training for the minor leagues: Easing into longer sleep intervals

Encouraging your baby to sleep longer at night is a common goal for new dads, and while it may seem challenging, there are effective ways to help your little teammate achieve more restful sleep. One practical approach is to gradually stretch the intervals between feedings as your baby grows. In the early days, it may feel like you're constantly feeding, but as your baby matures, they can consume more at each feeding, allowing for longer periods between meals. This helps your baby sleep for extended stretches, making the night feel more restful for both of you. It's like giving them a little more fuel in the tank so they can cruise through the night with fewer pit stops.

Another way to extend nighttime sleep is to introduce more structured naps during the day. Consistent nap times can help regulate your baby's sleep-wake cycle, making nighttime sleep more predictable and stabilizing your baby's internal clock. As you observe your baby's natural nap patterns, try to schedule them at regular intervals. This consistency helps prevent overtiredness, which can lead to restless nights. Gradually, as your baby becomes accustomed to these structured naps, you'll likely notice an improvement in their nighttime sleep quality and everyone will get a bit more shut-eye.

Babies are unpredictable, and what works one week might not work the next. Be prepared to adapt as your baby grows and changes. There will be nights when your baby sleeps peacefully and others when it feels like you're back to square one. It's important to recognize when adjustments are needed, perhaps tweaking nap times or feeding schedules to better align with your baby's current needs. Remember, there's no one-size-fits-all solution.

Sleep Pattern Tracker

You may want to start a sleep pattern tracker to help make sense of these unpredictable times. It can be as simple as jotting down when your baby sleeps and wakes in a notebook, or you might use a digital app to track your baby's sleep. Some good examples are Huckleberry, Glow Baby, and Baby Tracker. Features to look for in a great baby sleep tracker are sleep pattern analysis, sleep schedule suggestions, feeding tracking integration, white noise options, and multiple-user access. Keeping tabs on your newborn's sleep is like analyzing game stats—it gives you the insights you need to adjust your strategy. It also lets you identify any emerging patterns or preferences your baby might have. Over time, you'll notice trends that can guide you in creating a more structured sleep routine as your baby grows. Tracking these patterns will help you understand your baby's natural rhythms and offer reassurance that the sleepless nights contribute to their healthy development. Knowing when your baby tends to sleep more or less can also help you plan your day, ensuring you and your partner get the rest you need.

There are times when professional advice can be invaluable. If you consistently struggle with your baby's sleep, consulting a pediatrician or sleep consultant might provide the guidance you need. Persistent sleep issues can sometimes signal underlying concerns that require expert attention. These professionals can offer tailored advice, and perhaps suggest specific strategies or adjustments that can make a world of difference. Remember, seeking help is a sign of strength, not weakness. You're arming yourself with the knowledge and support needed to make informed decisions for your baby's well-being. Please remember that you're not alone. Countless dads have walked this path before you, and with perseverance and support, you'll soon find your rhythm.

As we wrap up this chapter, it's clear that sleep, or the lack of it, is a central theme in early parenthood. However, with the right strategies and support, you can help your whole family enjoy more restful nights. As you turn the page to the next chapter, we'll explore the nuances of keeping the romance alive with your loved one, an essential element in maintaining a strong, connected family unit.

8

Keeping the Spark Alive – Playing as a Team Off the Field

It's late at night, and the house is finally quiet. You and your wife are lying in bed, exhausted but unable to sleep. You turn to her, wanting to share a moment of connection, but your words and loving gestures seem lost in the fog of fatigue. In the stillness, you wonder how to keep the spark alive when your world feels turned upside down by the arrival of your bundle of joy. This chapter deals with rekindling romance and navigating the shifting dynamics of your relationship as you both step into parenthood's demanding roles.

Adjusting to the shifting team dynamics

It's common to fear that your relationship's dynamics will change with the birth of your child. You might worry that the strong connection you share with your wife or partner will be overshadowed by parenthood's new responsibilities. This is a concern many new dads face, as the arrival of a baby often shifts the focus from the couple to the baby and the family as a whole. Suddenly, the conversations that once revolved around weekend plans or shared hobbies now center on diaper brands, onesies, and sleep schedules. It's normal to feel apprehensive about this transition, as the new roles you both assume can sometimes feel overwhelming, leaving little room for nurturing your relationship.

Adjusting to this shift involves recognizing that change doesn't have to mean loss. While your relationship will evolve, it can grow stronger as you adapt to your new roles. It's important to acknowledge that both of you are experiencing this change, and it's okay to express your fears and insecurities. Open communication becomes your lifeline, allowing you to articulate how you feel and what you need from each other. By sharing these concerns, you validate your feelings and create a space where she can express hers. This mutual understanding can ease the anxiety of change, reminding you both that you're in this together.

Understanding that your partner might share similar worries can be reassuring. She, too, might feel concerned about maintaining your connection amidst the demands of caring for a newborn. It's vital to make time for each other, even in the midst of baby chaos. Reassure her that your relationship remains a priority. This doesn't mean grand gestures or elaborate plans; sometimes, small, everyday acts of kindness make the biggest difference. A simple hug, a cup of coffee made just as she likes it, or a note left on the fridge can reaffirm your commitment to each other. These gestures show that you're not just partners in parenting but also in life.

Keeping the fire burning

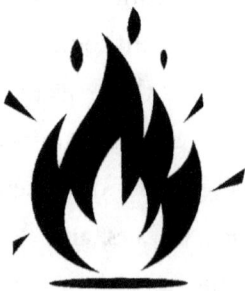

Intimacy usually takes a backseat in the daily grind of diaper changes and midnight feedings. Yet, maintaining a physical and emotional connection with your loved one is vital for a healthy, supportive relationship, especially during the transformative period after childbirth. The bond you share is the backbone that supports your relationship and therefore your entire family. Rebuilding intimacy may take time and patience as you adjust to new routines and responsibilities. However, you must prioritize this connection, as it acts as a source of strength and joy amidst the challenges of parenthood.

Expressing gratitude is a powerful way to keep the romantic connection alive. Acknowledging her efforts—soothing a fussy baby at 3 a.m. or managing household tasks—reinforces your appreciation for each other. Take a moment to thank her verbally for her contributions and recognize the hard work she's putting in. Write her love notes and leave them in unexpected places: a sweet message on the bathroom mirror or a text that pops up during her day can brighten her spirits and remind her of your love. Compliments can go a long way, even when you're both tired. Telling her she looks beautiful or praising her parenting skills can boost her confidence and reaffirm that she's cherished.

Romantic gestures don't have to be grand to be meaningful. Daily expressions of love and appreciation can make her feel special. Whether it's a surprise cup of her favorite coffee or planning a small outing, these acts show that you're thinking of her. Establishing small but meaningful traditions, like cooking dinner together once a week, can create lasting memories. Daily affection is another cornerstone of maintaining intimacy. Small gestures like hugs, kisses, holding hands, or sending a loving text during the day can lead to intimacy later. Acknowledge and appreciate each other's efforts as parents and partners. This shared recognition promotes a supportive environment where you feel valued and understood. In the chaos of caring for a newborn, these small acts help maintain a sense of normalcy and closeness.

Physical intimacy might take time to rekindle after childbirth, so be patient and gentle. Understand that it's okay for intimacy to evolve. Also, explore non-physical ways to reconnect, such as giving each other massages, sharing jokes, or having deep conversations about your future hopes and dreams while sharing a bubble bath. These interactions can reignite emotional closeness, laying the groundwork for physical intimacy to return naturally.

If adjusting to parenthood proves particularly challenging, seeking help can be incredibly beneficial. One option is to ask grandparents or trusted babysitters to come in regularly for a couple of hours, giving you both time to reconnect. This break will allow you to focus on each other, recharge, and maintain your relationship. Couples counseling or support groups can also provide a space to explore feelings and discover strategies to strengthen your bond. Don't hesitate to lean on family or friends for support—they can help create the space you need to keep the spark alive and strong.

Make time for the big plays

In the hustle of adjusting to life with a newborn, carving out time for just the two of you can feel like trying to score in overtime. Yet, prioritizing quality time away from the baby is essential for nurturing your relationship. It's easy to get caught up in the feedings, diaper changes, and sleep schedules, but remember that your partnership is the foundation of your family. Spending uninterrupted time together allows you to reconnect and focus on each other, away from the roles of mom and dad. You must find those timeouts in the middle of the chaos—moments to huddle up and remind each other why you started this game together in the first place. Scheduling regular date nights is a great way to carve out this time. While it might seem challenging with a newborn, it's not impossible. A few hours out at your favorite restaurant or a simple walk in the park can reignite the connection. If going out isn't feasible, transform your living room into a cozy retreat. Once the baby is asleep, light some candles and enjoy an ordered-in meal together at home. The setting doesn't have to be extravagant; it's the intention behind the action that counts. Sharing a meal without distractions allows for meaningful conversation and a chance to enjoy each other's company. Sometimes, it's the little things that bring you closer. After a long day, cuddling up on the couch and watching a show you both love can be incredibly comforting. It's a time to unwind and relax, enjoying the familiarity and warmth of each other's presence. Even a short episode of a sitcom can provide a much-needed break from the demands of parenthood and offer a moment to laugh and bond. Laughter is a powerful connector, reminding you of what brought you together. Share a quick cup of coffee or tea while the baby naps, or steal a few minutes to cuddle before bed, even if you're exhausted. These quick timeouts give you a chance to check in with each other and keep your connection strong.

Shared hobbies are another avenue to explore, especially if they've been neglected since the baby arrived. Revisit activities you both enjoy or find new ones to try together. If you love hiking, consider bringing the baby in a baby sling for a modified adventure. If you're into fitness, short workouts at home can be a fun way to stay active and spend time together. These shared experiences reinforce the idea that you're partners in more than just parenting; you're a team in life's adventures.

Planning for future activities can also be exciting. Talk about what you'd like to do once things settle down. It could be a trip you've always wanted to take or a professional game you're dying to see. Having something to look forward to keeps the spark alive and gives you a common goal. These conversations are a reminder that while things have changed, your shared dreams and desires remain.

Working together as a unit

When a baby joins the family, the dynamics shift, and teamwork becomes the glue that holds everything together. Parenting is like running plays as a team—you and your partner working together, supporting each other to create a strong and positive family environment. Effective teamwork involves more than just splitting duties; it's about creating a seamless balance where both of you feel valued. This collaboration nurtures a stronger relationship between you, setting a solid foundation for your growing family.

The benefits of teamwork in parenting extend beyond immediate tasks; they resonate through the emotional and psychological well-being of the entire family. A strong partnership sets a positive example for your children, showing them what a healthy, supportive relationship looks like. It provides a safety net during challenging times, ensuring neither parent feels overwhelmed or isolated. This sense of shared responsibility and mutual support strengthens the family bond, reducing stress and promoting happiness for everyone involved. When parents work together, they create an environment where children feel secure and loved, knowing they have a united team guiding them. It demonstrates that challenges are best faced as a unit, offering them a model for their interactions with others.

Building and strengthening your partnership requires intention and effort. Sharing parenting duties is one of the most effective ways to avoid burnout and ensure both partners feel supported. Co-parenting involves dividing tasks in a way that plays to each other's strengths but also allows for flexibility. Maybe one of you is better at soothing the baby to sleep, while the other excels at bath time. Recognizing these strengths and allowing room for growth helps distribute the workload evenly. Regarding household chores, tackling them as a team can prevent either partner from feeling overwhelmed. Create a system where weekly tasks are shared, alternating responsibilities to keep things fair and manageable.

Supporting each other's personal goals while co-parenting is also key for maintaining individuality within the partnership. Encourage each other to pursue hobbies or career aspirations, offering support and understanding as they do the same for you. This mutual encouragement strengthens your relationship and models the importance of personal growth and fulfillment for your children. It teaches them that while family is a priority, nurturing your own passions is equally important.

Celebrating teamwork and small victories as parents can reinforce your connection. Take a moment to acknowledge accomplishments, whether it's surviving the first week with a newborn or mastering a new parenting skill. These celebrations don't need to be elaborate—a simple toast over dinner or a high-five at the end of the day can boost morale and remind you of the progress you're making together.

Effective teamwork ensures that both partners feel involved and appreciated when handling parenthood's complexities. It's not just about dividing tasks but about supporting each other emotionally and practically. Working together creates a family dynamic that thrives on cooperation, love, and mutual respect. This partnership sets the stage for a nurturing environment where parents and children flourish, growing together with strength and resilience.

Clear communication: Strengthening the team

In the chaos of new parenthood, effective communication can literally keep your relationship intact. It's the bedrock upon which mutual understanding and support are built, especially when life seems consumed by the baby's needs. When both parents are on the same page through open communication, it builds a strong team that can handle whatever challenges come their way. Effective communication ensures that misunderstandings are minimized and both partners feel heard and valued. Try to connect on a deeper level by openly sharing your thoughts, fears, and aspirations.

Active listening is an integral part of this process. Try to truly listen—acknowledging her words without rushing to respond. Set aside distractions, make eye contact, and show empathy where appropriate. This exercise can transform dialogues into meaningful exchanges where you both feel truly understood. It promotes a sense of safety and trust, allowing both partners to express themselves freely without fear of judgment.

Non-verbal cues are equally powerful in communication. A simple touch on the shoulder, a hug, a warm smile, or a reassuring nod can speak volumes when words fall short. These cues often convey emotions that words cannot, offering comfort and support in moments of stress or uncertainty. They are easy reminders that you're in this together for the long haul. Being mindful of these non-verbal signals can deepen your connection, showing her you're present and engaged, even amid the chaos.

Open communication also involves discussing needs, concerns, and emotions honestly. You want to create a safe space where both partners can voice their feelings without fear of backlash. Sharing these emotions can prevent misunderstandings and resentment from building up over time. Whether expressing frustration over a sleepless night or sharing the joy of a baby's first smile, these conversations strengthen your connection. They allow you to cope with challenges together, supporting each other through the highs and lows.

As first mentioned in chapter one, an effective technique is to use "I" instead of "You" statements when communicating feelings. This approach shifts the focus from blame to personal experience, reducing defensiveness. For example, instead of saying, "You never help with the baby," try, "I feel overwhelmed when we don't share baby duties." This subtle change in phrasing opens the door for constructive dialogue, where solutions can be explored collaboratively. It encourages empathy and understanding, fostering a more harmonious relationship.

Incorporating regular check-ins over coffee or lunch can also enhance communication. Set aside time each week to discuss how you're feeling, what's working well, and what needs improvement. These check-ins create opportunities to address issues before they escalate, ensuring that both of you remain aligned. They're a chance to reconnect amidst the demands of parenting, reinforcing the partnership that brought you together. By prioritizing these moments, you're investing in the health and longevity of your relationship, ensuring that it remains strong and supportive.

Reconnecting and rebuilding after conflict

Even the strongest relationships face conflicts and sometimes fall short, especially when dealing with the challenges of new parenthood. Disagreements about parenting styles or household chores will arise, leaving both of you feeling distressed. However, these moments, though difficult, present opportunities for growth. Reconnecting after a conflict is vital for maintaining a resilient partnership. You want to repair the rift and reinforce your bond as quickly as possible.

Handling disagreements effectively requires a thoughtful approach. When tempers flare over parenting decisions or the division of chores, it's critical to approach the situation with a calm mindset. Step back and walk away for thirty minutes to clear your head and allow emotions to settle before diving into a discussion. Begin by acknowledging each other's perspectives, even if you don't entirely agree. This act of validation can diffuse tension and pave the way for more productive conversations. Consider setting aside a designated time to discuss contentious topics to ensure you are both in the right headspace. This structured approach can prevent minor issues from escalating into major conflicts and allow you to address concerns thoughtfully and constructively.

Forgiveness is so important when trying to move forward after an argument. Holding onto grudges creates emotional distance and erodes the trust and intimacy that form the foundation of your relationship. Instead, focus on letting go of past grievances and embracing the present. Forgiveness is a choice that requires empathy and a willingness to put pride aside and prioritize the health of your relationship. It's about acknowledging that you are both human and prone to mistakes and misunderstandings. By choosing to forgive, you create space for healing and growth, allowing your partnership to emerge stronger and more united. This practice of forgiveness promotes a culture of compassion and ensures that love remains at the core of your relationship.

Rebuilding emotional closeness after a disagreement is equally important. After resolving a conflict, take proactive steps to reconnect with your partner emotionally and physically. This might involve engaging in activities that bring you joy, simply spending quiet time together, or sharing intimacy. These moments of connection serve as reminders of the bond you share, reinforcing the love that brought you together in the first place. Consider establishing a ritual for after-conflict reconciliation, such as sharing a meal or going for a walk. These rituals can provide a sense of closure and allow you both to move forward with renewed commitment and understanding. By prioritizing these moments, you strengthen the emotional fabric of your relationship, ensuring that it remains resilient and robust.

Each conflict, while challenging, offers an opportunity for deeper understanding and connection. You need to transform friction into a force for good to shape a dynamic and enduring partnership. Reconnecting after conflict isn't just about resolving differences; it's about embracing the journey of growth and discovery together. As you navigate parenthood's complexities, remember that a strong relationship is your greatest asset. By promoting a culture of empathy, forgiveness, and reconnection, you lay the groundwork for a partnership that thrives amidst life's challenges. With each step forward, you build a future rooted in love, trust, and shared commitment.

9

Keeping Your Head in the Game – Emotional Health and Self-Care

Understanding fatherhood's highs and lows

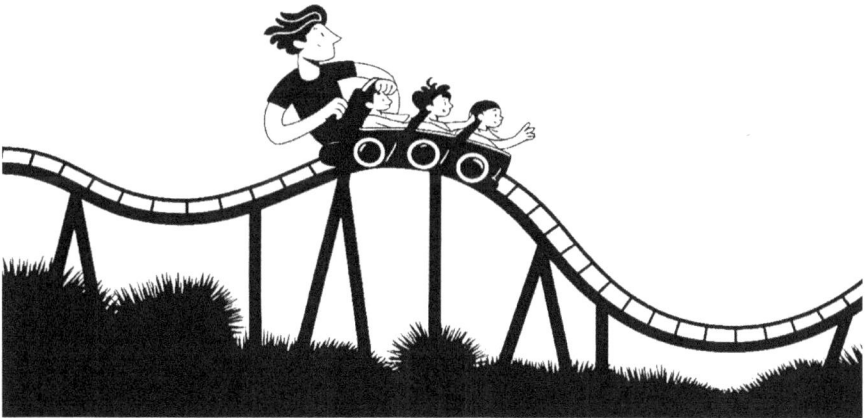

The first time you hold your newborn in your arms, it's as if the world stops. After that, being a dad can feel like an emotional rollercoaster, from elation and pride to a creeping anxiety about what lies ahead. You might find yourself marveling at your baby's first smile one moment and worrying about the utilities bill the next. Questions about affording diapers, saving for college, and balancing work commitments can weigh heavily on your mind. It's okay to feel anxious about these things. The main thing is acknowledging these feelings without letting them overshadow the joy of fatherhood. Recognizing that it's normal to experience a range of emotions can be liberating. It's important to remember that every dad goes through this; you're not the only one. It's a journey filled with highs and lows, and each emotion deserves a place in your experience of fatherhood.

You might not expect hormones to play a role in your season of fatherhood, but they do. When you become a dad, your testosterone levels can dip, which can influence your mood and emotional responses. This shift, while natural, can sometimes make you feel more vulnerable or irritable. It's similar to the hormonal changes that mothers experience, though less frequently discussed. Understanding these biological shifts can help you understand why you might feel off-kilter or more testy than usual. It's not just the lack of sleep or the new responsibilities—your body is adjusting to fatherhood in its own way.

When managing these emotional highs and lows, a few strategies can be game-changing. Practicing mindfulness and meditation can provide a sense of calm amidst the chaos. Taking even five minutes daily to focus on your breath or clear your mind can help you regain balance. Another powerful resource is connecting with other dads who understand what you're going through. Dad support groups offer a space to share experiences, swap tips, and find comfort in knowing other dads are dealing with similar challenges. These connections can prove to be invaluable, providing the camaraderie that helps you keep your footing when things get tough.

Open dialogue is a priority. Whether with your wife or a trusted friend, talking about your feelings can lighten the load. Expressing your fears or frustrations helps prevent them from festering. When you share your experiences, you pave the way for understanding and support. She too is likely dealing with her own emotional rollercoaster, and by sharing your thoughts, you encourage a partnership where both of you feel heard and supported. This open communication creates a foundation for a strong relationship, benefiting you, your partner, and your child.

Spotting and tackling postpartum depression: A game plan for support

You may be sitting on the couch, your newborn finally asleep in the crib, but instead of feeling peace, you're hit with an unexpected wave of sadness. It's not just exhaustion from sleepless nights; it feels more profound and more persistent. Paternal postpartum depression (PPPD) is a reality that many new dads face, though it's often whispered about rather than openly discussed. Mothers aren't the only ones who are affected by postpartum depression. You might feel persistently irritable or disconnected, or perhaps you've lost interest in activities you once loved. These are not just fleeting "baby blues." They can be signs of PPPD, a condition that affects about 25% of new fathers, even if only a fraction seek help. This depression can manifest as withdrawal from family and friends, a lack of energy, or changes in sleep and appetite. It might even lead to aggressive behavior or substance abuse if left unaddressed. Recognizing these symptoms is a vital first step toward finding balance again.

Addressing PPPD is often complicated by cultural norms. Many men feel pressure to be the family's rock, to push through without showing weakness. It's a stigma that discourages seeking help, rooted in outdated notions of masculinity. Yet, acknowledging the struggle is not a sign of weakness but strength. It shows you're taking charge of your mental health for your sake and your family's. Breaking the silence around paternal mental health issues is essential. The more we talk about it, the more we normalize seeking support, creating a culture where dads feel empowered to reach out without fear of judgment. Remember, you're not the first one to feel like this. I've been there, and there's no shame in seeking help.

There are numerous resources available to help you find support. Connecting with mental health professionals is a vital step. They can offer personalized guidance and treatment options through therapy or medication. Many therapists specialize in men's mental health and understand the unique challenges faced by new dads. Support groups for fathers can also offer a lifeline. These groups provide a space to share experiences and strategies and to find camaraderie with other dads going through similar challenges. It's a reminder that you're not navigating this path by yourself—there's a community ready to support you. Online resources and hotlines can also provide immediate support and information.

Early intervention is key. Addressing symptoms sooner rather than later can have profound benefits for both you and your family. By seeking help early, you're improving your well-being and contributing to a healthier family environment. You're showing that caring for one's mental health is a priority, not an afterthought. Embracing this mindset can lead to stronger family bonds and a more fulfilling parenting experience.

For reference, below is a comprehensive list of PPPD symptoms.

Paternal Postpartum Depression Symptoms:

Emotional Symptoms:

- Persistent Sadness – Feeling down, hopeless, or empty most of the time.
- Increased Irritability or Anger – Short temper, frustration, or increased conflict with others.
- Feelings of Guilt or Shame – Believing you are a "bad" father or failing as a provider.
- Emotional Numbness – Feeling detached from your baby, partner, or life in general.
- Loss of Interest – No longer enjoying activities you once found pleasurable.
- Anxiety or Excessive Worry – Fear about your baby's well-being, financial responsibilities, or relationship changes.
- Mood Swings – Experiencing frequent emotional ups and downs.
- Feelings of Helplessness – Believing that nothing you do can make things better.

Cognitive Symptoms:

- Difficulty Concentrating – Trouble focusing on work or everyday tasks.
- Indecisiveness – Difficulty making even simple decisions.
- Intrusive Thoughts – Having disturbing thoughts about harm coming to the baby or yourself.
- Negative Self-Perception – Feeling inadequate or believing you are not a good father.
- Rumination – Repeatedly going over worries, fears, or mistakes in your mind.

Behavioral Symptoms:

- Withdrawal from Family and Friends – Avoiding social interactions and isolating yourself.
- Avoidance of the Baby – Reluctance to hold, care for, or interact with the child.
- Increased Work Hours – Using work as an escape from home responsibilities.
- Substance Use – Increased use of alcohol, nicotine, or drugs to cope with emotions.
- Risky or Reckless Behavior – Engaging in dangerous activities or making impulsive decisions.
- Lack of Motivation – Struggling to complete daily tasks or responsibilities.
- Increased Conflict with Partner – More arguments, irritability, or resentment towards your spouse or co-parent.

Physical Symptoms:

- Fatigue – Constant exhaustion, even with adequate sleep.
- Sleep Disturbances – Insomnia, trouble falling asleep, or sleeping too much.
- Appetite Changes – Eating significantly more or less than usual.
- Headaches or Muscle Pain – Increased physical discomfort without a clear medical cause.
- Lowered Libido – Reduced sexual interest or performance issues.
- Weakened Immune System – More frequent illnesses or prolonged recovery times.

Severe Symptoms (Indicating a Need for Immediate Help):

- Suicidal Thoughts – Thinking about self-harm or believing your family would be better off without you.
- Homicidal Thoughts – Thoughts of harming others, including your baby or partner.
- Complete Emotional Detachment – Feeling completely disconnected from reality, family, or life in general.
- Severe Aggression or Violence – Physical aggression, abusive tendencies, or explosive outbursts.

When to Seek Help:

If you experience several of these symptoms for two weeks or longer, professional help should be sought. Therapy, support groups, lifestyle changes, and in some cases, medication can help manage PPPD.

Staying in the zone: Pro tips for managing stress

Work-Life Balance and Time Management

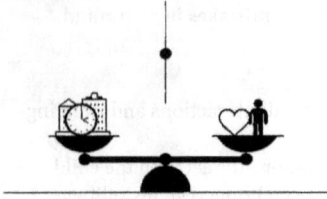

Let's talk about stress, that persistent companion that often tags along when you become a new dad. You're juggling work, family, and personal time, and it can feel like you're in a constant balancing act. Work demands might clash with family time, leaving you torn between meeting deadlines and being present at home. The pressure to excel in your career while ensuring you're there for those first smiles and giggles is real. This balancing act can impact your emotional well-being, making it necessary to find ways to manage these competing demands. You must establish an up-front routine that accommodates work and family life, allowing you to be effective in both areas without burning out. Set firm boundaries between work and personal time, perhaps by dedicating specific hours to family activities or ensuring you disconnect from work emails during family time. This separation will allow you to be fully present in each aspect of your life, reducing stress and enhancing your overall well-being.

It's easy to feel like there aren't enough hours in the day to balance everything. One practical strategy is to prioritize tasks and break them into manageable chunks. Use a planner or digital calendar to organize your day, allocating specific times for work, family, and personal activities. This structure can help you maintain focus and make the most of your time. Remember, it's okay to delegate tasks or ask for help when needed, whether sharing household duties at home or seeking assistance from family and friends. By setting realistic goals and embracing flexibility, you can create a balanced schedule that supports your responsibilities and well-being.

Financial Pressures

Financial pressures add another layer of stress, as providing for a growing family can feel overwhelming. You may worry about budgeting for baby supplies, planning for future expenses, and maintaining financial security. These concerns are valid but managing them is possible with careful planning. Start by creating a detailed budget that outlines your monthly expenses and identifies areas where you can save. Prioritize essential costs and explore cost-effective options for non-essentials. Being proactive about your finances can alleviate the anxiety of financial responsibilities. It's also helpful to periodically review and adjust your budget as your family's needs change, ensuring you stay on track and avoid unexpected financial strain.

Seeking Support

Seeking support is another crucial aspect of stress management. Don't be afraid to ask for help, whether talking to a mental health professional, joining a support group, or simply confiding in a close friend. Sharing your experiences and concerns with others can provide valuable perspective and reassurance. It's a reminder that you're not alone in dealing with the challenges of fatherhood and that seeking support is a sign of strength, not weakness. By taking proactive steps to manage stress, you can cultivate a healthier, more balanced approach to fatherhood, allowing you to enjoy the journey and be the best dad you can be.

Playing defense against the fear of losing your freedom

When you become a dad, one of the most significant changes you might face is the shift in how you spend your time. It can feel like the freedom you once had to pursue hobbies, hang out with friends, or make spontaneous plans is slipping away. It's a genuine concern for many new dads who grapple with the fear of losing personal freedom. You might worry about saying goodbye to weekend fishing trips, late-night gaming sessions, or even the ability to decide on a whim to grab a beer with a buddy. These activities aren't mere pastimes; they're part of what makes you, well, you. The thought of losing them can feel overwhelming.

But here's the thing: While your schedule will definitely change, it doesn't mean you have to give up everything you love. You'll just need to find a new balance. Personal time is necessary for your sanity and for being the best dad you can be. Think of it as recharging your batteries. Scheduling regular personal downtime can help you maintain a sense of self during the wild game of parenthood. Maybe it's setting aside an hour on Sunday afternoons for your favorite hobby or penciling in a monthly poker night with the guys. These recovery moments are like little lifelines, keeping you grounded and connected to who you are outside of being a dad.

Engaging in activities that bring you joy isn't indulgent; it's necessary. Whether taking a jog, going to the gym, or tinkering with your car, these pursuits offer a much-needed mental break. They allow you to return to your family refreshed and more present. Communicating about these needs is key, as well as ensuring you support each other's personal time. After all, she might also crave moments with her girlfriends, and working together to accommodate this can strengthen your partnership. Make a conscious effort to carve out time for these hobbies and social interactions, even if it means shorter or less frequent outings.

Connecting with friends is another critical component of maintaining personal freedom. Those friendships you've nurtured over the years shouldn't fade away just because you're a parent now. Sure, you might not be able to meet up as often or stay out as late, but finding creative ways to stay in touch can keep those relationships alive. Maybe it's a quick catch-up over lunch during the workweek or a virtual hangout after the kids are asleep. These interactions will remind you that you're still part of a broader social circle, offering support and camaraderie.

The idea of spontaneous decisions might seem like a distant memory when you're knee-deep in diapers and feeding schedules. But don't write off spontaneity entirely. It might just look a little different now. Perhaps it's planning a surprise picnic for your family or taking a last-minute drive to your favorite spot. Allowing room for these unplanned moments can add a touch of excitement to your routine, proving that parenthood doesn't have to mean the end of spontaneity. It just shifts in focus, adapting to include the little one you've welcomed into your life. So, pack the baby bag, strap your family in, and head on out!

Deflecting unsolicited parenting advice like a pro

You're at a family gathering, proudly holding your newborn, when Aunt Karen swoops in with an onslaught of advice on how to "properly" hold the baby. Next, Uncle Chad chimes in about the merits of old-school parenting techniques, leaving you wondering if he's ever even changed a diaper. As a new dad, you'll quickly realize unsolicited parenting advice is as common as sleepless nights. Often, the loudest voices come from family members who cling to outdated views, convinced that the way they did things is the only way. Their intentions might be good, but it can feel overwhelming (and a little irritating) when you're trying to find your own parenting style. Then there are well-meaning friends, perhaps childless themselves, who offer differing opinions based on what they've read or heard. The sheer volume of advice can leave you questioning your instincts, adding unnecessary pressure to an already challenging time.

When faced with a tidal wave of advice, the key is to respond like a pro without sparking conflict. Acknowledging the advice with a polite nod or a simple "Thanks, we'll consider that" can make a powerhouse impact. It shows appreciation without committing you to any particular course of action. Another tactic is to skillfully redirect the conversation to your parenting choices. You might say, "That's interesting, but we've decided to try this approach," and then shift the subject to something less contentious. This strategy preserves relationships and reinforces your role as the decision-maker in your child's life. Remember, you and your wife or partner are the ultimate authorities on your baby, and your approach is valid, even if it doesn't align with others' views.

Setting boundaries is another way to manage external influences on your parenting journey. It's okay to politely let people know when their advice isn't wanted or needed. Establishing clear boundaries can help prevent unwanted opinions from occupying too much mental space. You might say something like, "We appreciate your input, but we're handling it differently." This straightforward approach can help protect your peace and maintain your focus on your family's unique needs. Boundaries don't only involve keeping unwanted advice at bay; they also create a space where your parenting choices are respected and valued. By establishing limits, you create an environment that supports your growth as a father, allowing you to handle parenthood's challenges with clarity and conviction.

Confidence in your personal parenting decisions is fundamental. You need to trust your instincts. You've spent nine months preparing, researching, and discussing plans with your wife or partner. You're equipped with the knowledge and instincts necessary to make the best choices for your child. Sure, there will be moments of doubt and mistakes—that's normal—but it's essential to remember that being an awesome father isn't about perfection. It's about being present, loving, and willing to learn. As you grow more comfortable in your dad role, your confidence will naturally increase, making it easier to tune out the noise and focus on what truly matters.

Footing the bill for the team

The thought of financial preparedness can keep any new dad up at night. The cost of raising a child is enormous, and looming uncertainties about managing these expenses can weigh heavily on your mind. You might find yourself crunching numbers repeatedly, trying to figure out how to fit new expenses into an already tight budget. When your little one arrives, a slew of new expenses will pile up. Below is a list of everyday family expenses to consider and plan for as your baby arrives, plus a few helpful strategies to help keep your costs in check.

Expenses to Consider:

- Baby supplies and gear (diapers, formula, creams, shampoos/lotions, blankets, swaddlers, baby slings, car seats, etc.)

- Clothing and toys will become regular purchases as your baby grows out of everything faster than you can keep up.

- Setting up a nursery is another significant expense, whether purchasing a crib, a changing table, or simply decorating the room with a cozy theme.

- Food expenses will grow as your baby transitions from milk to solids, and that's just the beginning.

- Medical expenses, including hospital delivery costs, prenatal care, and pediatric visits, can quickly add up. Checking your insurance coverage is crucial to understanding what's covered and what you'll need to pay out of pocket.

- Health insurance plays a vital role in managing medical costs. Confirm your prenatal, delivery, and postpartum care coverage, and plan to add your baby to your health insurance after birth.

- Consider contributing to a Flexible Spending Account (FSA) or Health Savings Account (HSA) to cover medical costs with pre-tax dollars, reducing the financial burden.

- Planning for parental leave is another essential consideration. Review your employer's policies regarding paid or unpaid leave and save enough to cover any gaps in income during this period.

- Estimating childcare costs early on can help you prepare for this significant expense. Research daycare options, join waiting lists, and consider flexible work arrangements that might reduce future childcare costs. Whether considering daycare, hiring a nanny, or relying on family help, these options require financial planning.

- Life insurance and estate planning become more critical as you consider securing your child's future.

- Establishing a college fund, like a 529 account, might be something you haven't even considered yet, but it's worth planning for early on.

Financial Planning Strategies

Budgeting and money-saving strategies become your allies in coping with these financial challenges. Start by creating a detailed baby budget that outlines all potential expenses. Research typical costs for baby essentials and factor in medical expenses, ensuring you have a clear picture of what to expect. Adjust your lifestyle to accommodate these new costs, perhaps cutting back on dining out or subscriptions to free up funds.

Building an emergency fund is another crucial step. Aim to save enough to cover three to six months of living expenses, providing a cushion for unexpected situations like job loss or medical emergencies. Automate savings to make regular contributions to this fund, ensuring it grows steadily over time.

Daily expenses will undoubtedly increase with a baby in the house. Diapers and formulas are recurring costs, so look for discounts, coupons, or subscription services to save money. Stock up on baby supplies gradually to spread out expenses, and budget for increased utilities and groceries as your household grows.

Relatives and friends often want to buy gifts for the new baby, and it's helpful to have a list of items you need ready if they ask for suggestions. That way, instead of Grandma buying yet another useless giant teddy bear, you can suggest that she buys a crib, bottle sterilizer, or baby clothing. This will take the pressure off you to provide every single item and will give loved ones the satisfaction of feeling that they're contributing something truly useful.

Tackling debt is another critical step in financial planning. Pay down high-interest debt to free up funds for baby expenses and consider refinancing existing loans to lower monthly payments.

Updating financial documents is an intimidating but vital task. Create or update your will, name a guardian for your child, and establish a plan for managing assets. Adjust beneficiaries on life insurance and retirement accounts to include your child and ensure both parents have adequate life insurance to protect the family's financial future.

10

Stepping Up to the Plate – Owning the Modern Dad Role

You're standing in your living room, surrounded by baby toys, a stack of parenting books, and a tired but happy mom. It hits you—you're not just a bystander in this parenting gig but a central player. The role of a father has dramatically evolved, and today, it involves being actively engaged, nurturing, and present. Gone are the days when dads were merely the breadwinners, distant from the day-to-day parenting grind. Now, fathers are rolling up their sleeves, diving into diaper duty, and attending school functions and field trips with pride.

Changing coaches: Out with the old, in with the new

Historically, fathers were seen as the disciplinarians and providers, while mothers took on the nurturing roles. This division of labor was born out of necessity and cultural norms but left many dads feeling disconnected from their children. Fast forward to today, and you'll notice a significant shift. Economic changes, such as the increased participation of women in the workforce, have altered these roles. Fathers are now more involved in caregiving, a socially accepted and encouraged change. Men are embracing this transformation by taking paternity leave, attending parenting classes, and engaging in the everyday care of their kids.

Active fatherhood brings a multitude of benefits, both for your children and your family as a whole. We know that when dads are involved, children tend to have better emotional health and improved social skills. They develop a sense of security, knowing they have a loving father who is there for them. Statistics show that kids with engaged dads perform better in school and develop a stronger sense of identity. By being present, you're strengthening family bonds and contributing to a stable, secure home environment. Your involvement can also lead to improved co-parenting, as you work together, sharing responsibilities and supporting each other.

Modern dads are redefining what it means to be a father, and it's exciting to see the different ways this manifests. Take, for example, attending parent-teacher conferences or volunteering at school events. Traditionally, this role was only performed by moms. Historically, men very rarely participated in their children's school functions. However, in today's society, the modern dad is showing up and getting involved. Being a part of school activities shows your kids that you value them and their education and allows you to be an integral part of their academic journey.

Flexible work arrangements are another way dads are stepping up. More companies today recognize the importance of work-life balance, allowing fathers to adjust their schedules to be more present at home. This flexibility can make a significant difference, allowing you to bond with your newborn during those precious early months.

Finally, embracing modern fatherhood means creating your own path. There's no one-size-fits-all approach to being a dad. You need to find what works for you and your family and align your parenting with your values and needs. Maybe you value quality time over quantity or are passionate about teaching your kids through shared activities. Whatever your approach, the key is to be intentional and engaged. Embrace the role, relish the moments, and remember that your presence is your greatest gift to your children.

Sharing the load: Crafting a balanced team

Imagine tackling parenting like a two-player game where both players are equally engaged and committed. It's about finding that sweet spot where responsibilities are shared, and partners feel supported and valued. The idea of equality in parenting is not simply a modern trend; it's necessary for creating a harmonious household. When you both divide household chores, it ensures that no one feels overburdened. Whether it's managing laundry, doing the dishes, or handling grocery shopping, splitting these tasks can prevent burnout and promote teamwork. Similarly, shared cooking responsibilities can turn meal prep from a mundane chore into an opportunity to bond and collaborate.

Bedtime routines are another area where shared responsibilities can make a significant impact. When you take turns putting the kids to bed, it gives the other parent a break and helps the children form bonds with both parents. This routine can include reading stories, tucking in, or simply talking about the day. Equal participation in childcare duties, such as changing diapers and bathing, further strengthens the partnership. When both parents are involved in these everyday tasks, it sends a powerful message to your children about teamwork and cooperation.

In the traditional role, dads unfortunately got the bad rap of being the primary disciplinarian. Being equal partners in discipline is another important aspect of this balance. Presenting a united front when setting rules and boundaries is critical as it ensures consistency and clear boundaries for your children. It also models positive behavior, showing them the value of collaboration and equality. When both parents are on the same page, it creates a stable and secure environment for everyone.

As mentioned earlier, attending parent-teacher conferences together and helping with homework also ensures that you're engaged in your child's education, reinforcing the idea that both parents are equally invested in their development. The same goes for your child's extra-curricular activities – get involved and be present!

To help manage family schedules and responsibilities, a shared family calendar can be a lifesaver, helping you manage schedules and responsibilities. It's a simple tool that informs everyone about important dates and appointments. Alternating duties and rotating responsibilities can keep things fair and prevent one parent from feeling overwhelmed. Regular check-ins are essential to adjust responsibilities, especially as family dynamics change over time.

Flexibility is key as family roles and responsibilities evolve. Life with kids is ever-changing, and what worked last month might not work the next. Being open to change and adapting to the current situation is essential. This adaptability ensures your partnership remains strong and responsive to your family's needs.

Strategizing for the future: Long-term parenting goals

Imagine yourself a few years down the road. Your child's first school play is coming up, and they're practicing their lines in the living room with excitement and a hint of nerves in their eyes. Moments like these remind us of the importance of setting long-term parenting goals. Defining what kind of parent and role model you want to be isn't just about today or tomorrow; it's about the legacy you leave behind. Start by thinking about your core family values. Is it kindness, integrity, or curiosity you want to instill in your children? These values will guide your decisions and actions about parenting, providing a compass as your family grows.

Educational aspirations play a significant role in shaping your child's future. Maybe you envision them thriving in a specific academic field, or perhaps you hope they find joy in lifelong learning, regardless of the path they choose. These aspirations don't have to be rigid. Instead, they should reflect your values, such as resilience, creativity, or perseverance. Discuss these hopes and dreams, ensuring you're both aligned in your vision. This shared understanding creates a unified front as you tackle issues like what schools to choose and what colleges to save funds for.

Working towards these long-term objectives requires more than wishful thinking; it demands action and commitment. Set aside time for regular goal-setting sessions with your loved one. These sessions can be a space to dream, plan, and adjust your parenting strategies. During these discussions, you might create a family mission statement—a guiding document that captures your collective values and priorities. It doesn't have to be formal or complex. A simple statement encapsulating what matters to you can be a strong anchor.

Life, as we know, loves to throw curveballs. This is why adaptability is fundamental. As your children grow, their needs and interests will evolve. Your long-term goals should be flexible enough to accommodate these changes without losing sight of your core values. Embrace this fluidity, knowing it allows your family to grow and thrive in an ever-changing world.

Regular reflection on your parenting impact is a practice that will keep you grounded. Take time to evaluate, considering what's working and what might need a tweak. Are you living up to the values you set out to embody? How are your actions influencing your child's development? These reflections can be sobering but are essential for growth. They remind you that parenting isn't about perfection but progress and presence. Adjustments are not signs of failure but opportunities to refine your approach, ensuring you remain the steady, loving presence your children need.

Building your dad team: Creating a strong support squad

Imagine being part of a group where everyone gets it. You're not just another dad; you're part of a community that listens, shares advice, and has your back when parenting feels like a never-ending rollercoaster. Connecting with other dads can be a game changer. It provides emotional and practical support, helping you get through fatherhood's ups and downs. By sharing experiences and advice, you'll gain insights into different approaches and solutions to common challenges. You're not alone in this, and sometimes, all it takes is a conversation with a buddy who's been there to make things clearer. Organizing regular dad meet-ups or hangouts is an excellent way to grow these connections. It's not just the kids who benefit from these outings; dads get to bond, share stories, and even vent about the things only other dads would understand.

Finding and building a dad community might initially seem tough, but it's easier than you think. Start by joining local parenting groups or online forums. These spaces are goldmines of collective wisdom and camaraderie. You might be surprised at how willing other men are to share their experiences and offer support. Participating in kids' activities and school events can connect you with other dads with similar interests and challenges. Whether volunteering for a school event or cheering from the sidelines at a high school football game, these interactions lay the groundwork for friendships.

Joining dad-friendly fitness groups is another great option. Whether it's a weekend hike or a casual basketball game, these activities provide a perfect mix of exercise and male bonding. Community events geared towards families are also solid opportunities to meet other dads. And don't underestimate the power of organizing a dads' night out! Sometimes, a low-key dinner or trip to a local sporting event can be just what you need to recharge and connect.

Collaboration and resource sharing are at the heart of a strong dad community. Everyone benefits when you pool resources, whether it's knowledge about the best local pediatrician or tips for balancing work and family life. This collective approach can make the challenges of fatherhood feel less overwhelming. Dads can trade plays, from babysitting substitutions to parenting pro tips, creating a network that supports each member. Beyond practical tips, these communities facilitate a culture of support and encouragement. Motivating one another and celebrating individual and collective successes strengthens bonds and builds confidence. It's about lifting one another up, knowing that together, you're better equipped to handle whatever fatherhood throws your way.

Leading by example: Being the MVP your kid looks up to

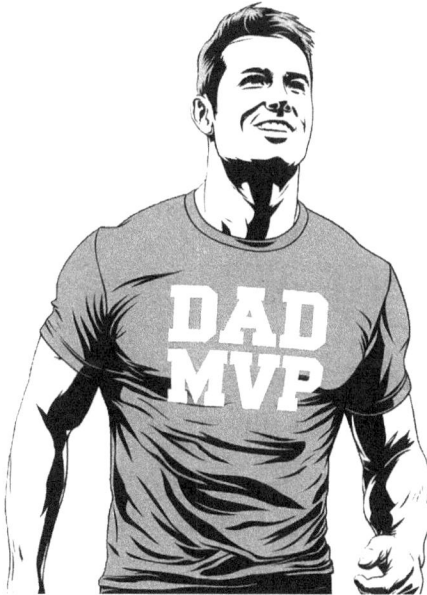

The impact of your behavior on your child is profound. Children are like sponges, soaking up everything they see and hear. They watch how you react to challenges, how you interact with others, and even how you handle stress. Children mirror their parents. Your actions and attitudes set a framework for them to understand the world and their place in it. Demonstrating kindness and empathy in your daily interactions teaches them the importance of compassion. When you show patience with a cashier or offer a helping hand to a neighbor, you're modeling behaviors they'll likely copy. These small, everyday moments don't go unnoticed by your child and leave a lasting impression.

Positive role modeling goes beyond being kind. It's also about making solid health choices, like grabbing a salad instead of a fast-food burger or hitting the pavement for a jog instead of crashing on the couch. These choices teach your child about self-care and the value of maintaining health.

When conflicts arise, handling them with calmness and respect, without resorting to yelling or blaming others, shows them how to resolve disagreements constructively. Collaborating as a team on family decisions further illustrates cooperation and compromise, which are fundamental skills for any relationship.

Managing stress by using healthy coping mechanisms, whether through mindfulness, exercise, or simply talking about your feelings, sets an example of emotional resilience. Apologizing and forgiving when necessary shows them humility and the importance of maintaining relationships.

Teaching responsibility and accountability is important too. Whether cleaning up after yourself or sticking to commitments, these actions speak volumes. Demonstrating a strong work ethic and an enthusiasm for lifelong learning encourages them to value education and hard work.

Get involved in community service activities, like volunteering at a local shelter or food pantry, demonstrates the significance of generosity and giving back. Showcasing gratitude and positivity, even on tough days, helps them appreciate life's small joys. Teaching financial responsibility, like saving for a rainy day, paired with financial generosity, such as donating to an important cause or charity, offers a balanced view of money.

Whether obeying traffic laws or listening to teachers, respect for rules and authority lays the groundwork for understanding the importance of societal structures.

Consistency is key. It's not enough to demonstrate these values occasionally. Children need to see them regularly to understand that they're not just ideals but a way of life in your family. This consistency builds trust and security, reinforcing the lessons you're imparting. Over time, these values will become ingrained in your children, shaping their character and guiding their choices later in life.

Self-reflection is a necessary exercise for any role model. Continually strive for personal growth and development. Set personal goals for improvement, whether it's becoming more patient or learning a new skill. Seeking feedback from family members can provide insights into how you can enhance your parenting skills. It's a journey of growth, not just for your child's sake but for your own. As you work on yourself, you're not only becoming a better dad but also a better person. And in doing so, you're giving your child a front-row seat to the self-improvement process and the rewards it brings.

Conclusion

As you wrap up *Dad Rookie: The Game-Changing Pregnancy Guide for First-Time Dads*, I want to call a quick time-out and reflect on the rookie season we've been tackling together. This guide was designed to equip you, as a first-time dad, with the tools, strategies, and confidence to take on the incredible adventure of fatherhood like a pro. From figuring out the ins and outs of pregnancy to nailing the basics of newborn care, you have a solid game plan to guide you through these key moments.

Throughout this guide, we broke down the trimesters of pregnancy, giving you the inside scoop on your baby's growth and the changes your partner goes through. We covered practical tips for being a solid teammate—like showing up for prenatal appointments and setting up a stress-free home base. The sections on bonding with your baby spotlighted key plays like skin-to-skin contact, tummy time, and interactive moments to build that winning connection early on.

Key takeaways include knowing the impact of your role, keeping open communication with your wife or partner, and the necessity of being actively involved in your baby's life. These are the pillars that will support you as you grow into your new role. Remember, empathy and patience are your best MVPs–they'll help you emotionally support your loved one and your baby.

Now, the real work begins. Take the pro tips, checklists, and strategies laid out here and apply them to your daily parenting game. Step into your new dad role with confidence and bring your A-game every day. The tips and tools provided are your stepping stones to becoming the father you aspire to be.

Fatherhood is a continuous learning experience. Stay curious and keep seeking knowledge. Parenting communities and resources are invaluable. They provide support, camaraderie, and a wealth of information. Don't hesitate to lean on them as you traverse the challenges and joys of raising your child. Staying engaged will elevate your fatherhood game and ensure you remain a positive force in your child's life.

Modern dads are changing the parenting playbook. Your hands-on, supportive presence is an essential influence. You play a critical role in your child's development and well-being, and your involvement creates a loving, secure environment where your child can thrive.

I want to give a big shout-out to you for choosing this book as your go-to guide. Thanks for being part of the team on this fatherhood journey. Remember, you're not out there playing solo—every challenge you face and every win you score is proof of your love and dedication as a dad. Just know there's a whole league of dads out there, grinding through the same highs and lows of fatherhood with you.

As you close this book, hold onto the knowledge and insights you've gained. Trust yourself and the bonds you are building with your child and new family. Fatherhood is like stepping into the championship game—one of the most rewarding experiences life throws your way. Dive in with everything you've got, and trust in yourself that you now have the skills and confidence to tackle parenting challenges like a true pro. Welcome to fatherhood—you're ready to nail it!

References

American College of Obstetricians and Gynecologists. Sample Birth Plan Template. https://www.acog.org/womens-health/health-tools/sample -birth-plan.

American Psychological Association. The changing role of the modern-day father. American Psychological Association. https://www.apa.org/pi/families/resources/changing-father#:~:text=I n%20summary%2C%20the%20modern%20day,remaining%20a%20pe rmanent%20and%20loving.

Bay, K., & Mortensen, O. (2023, March). The effect of antenatal education on expectant fathers. Journal of Family Studies. https://pmc.ncbi.nlm .nih.gov/articles/PMC9944450/.

BBC Tiny Happy People. New dads' mental health advice. BBC. https:/ /www.bbc.co.uk/tiny-happy-people/articles/zb7svk7.

Better Health Channel. Typical sleep behaviour (1) – Newborns 0 to 3 months. Victoria State Government. https://www.betterhealth.vic.go v.au/health/healthyliving/typical-sleep-behaviour-nb-0-3-months.

Carlson, M. J., & Meyer, D. R. (2018). The increasing diversity and complexity of family structures. Journal of Marriage and Family, 80(4), 823-839. https://pmc.ncbi.nlm.nih.gov/articles/PMC6124501/.

Carroll, A. (2020, April 15). How men's bodies change when they become fathers. The New York Times. https://www.nytimes.com/2020/04/1 5/parenting/baby/fatherhood-mens-bodies.html.

Cleveland Clinic. Preparing for fatherhood: Guide for new dads. Cleveland Clinic. https://health.clevelandclinic.org/preparing-for -fatherhood.

Cleveland Clinic. The benefits of reading to babies. Cleveland Clinic. https://health.clevelandclinic.org/the-benefits-of-reading-to-b abies.

Colorado State University. (2023, April 10). Increased expectations for fathers expose lack of support for dads. Colorado State University Source. https://chhs.source.colostate.edu/dadspace/.

Coming Home Magazine.Your complete babyproofing checklist. Coming Home Magazine. https://www.cominghomemag.com/fea tured-articles/babyproofing-checklist.

Gharaibeh, M. & Oweis, A. (2019, September). Couvade syndrome among Jordanian expectant fathers. Journal of Prenatal and Perinatal Psychology and Health, 34(1). https://pmc.ncbi.nlm.nih.gov/a rticles/PMC6771218/.

Gidget Foundation. How to manage the stress of becoming a new dad. Gidget Foundation. https://www.gidgetfoundation.org.au/fact-sh eets/how-to-manage-the-stress-of-becoming-a-new-dad.

HealthyChildren.org. How to calm a fussy baby: Tips for parents & caregivers. American Academy of Pediatrics. https://www.healthychildren.org/English/ages-stages/baby/ crying-colic/Pages/Calming-A-Fussy-Baby.aspx.

HealthyChildren.org. Swaddling: Is it safe for your baby? American Academy of Pediatrics. https://www.healthychildren.org/English/ ages-stages/baby/diapers-clothing/Pages/Swaddling-Is-it-Safe.aspx.

Inova Newsroom. (2019, June). Stress management for dads: How your mental health impacts your kids. Inova Newsroom. https://www.inovanewsroom.org/expert-commentary/2019/06/str ess-management-for-dads-how-your-mental-health-impacts-your-ki ds/.

KidCentral TN. Involved fathers provide key benefits to kids. KidCentral TN. https://www.kidcentraltn.com/support/full-family-support/involved-fathers-provide-key-benefits-to-kids.html.

Mayo Clinic Staff. Colic - Diagnosis & treatment. Mayo Clinic. https://www.mayoclinic.org/diseases-conditions/colic/diagnosis-treatment/drc-20371081.

Mayo Clinic Staff. Fetal development: The 1st trimester. Mayo Clinic. https://www.mayoclinic.org/healthy-lifestyle/pregnancy-week-by-week/in-depth/prenatal-care/art-20045302.

Mayo Clinic Staff. Fetal development: The 2nd trimester. Mayo Clinic. https://www.mayoclinic.org/healthy-lifestyle/pregnancy-week-by-week/in-depth/fetal-development/art-20046151.

Mayo Clinic Staff. 3rd trimester pregnancy: What to expect. Mayo Clinic. https://www.mayoclinic.org/healthy-lifestyle/pregnancy-week-by-week/in-depth/pregnancy/art-20046767.

Motherhood Center. Co-parenting 101: How new dads can support their partner. Motherhood Center. https://www.motherhoodcenter.com/how-new-dads-can-support-their-partner/.

Nanit. Hospital bag checklist for dad: 18 must-have items. Nanit. https://www.nanit.com/blogs/parent-confidently/hospital-bag-checklist.

Nationwide Children's Hospital. How to bathe your baby. Nationwide Children's Hospital. https://www.nationwidechildrens.org /family-resources-education/health-wellness-and-safety-resources/helping-hands/bathing-your-baby.

Nationwide Children's Hospital. Nursery safety. Nationwide Children's Hospital. https://www.nationwidechildrens.org/ research/areas-of-research/center-for-injury-research-and-policy/injury-topics/home-safety/nursery-safety.

Nationwide Children's Hospital. Safe sleep practices for babies. Nationwide Children's Hospital. https://www.nationwidechildrens.org/f

amily-resources-education/health-wellness-and-safety-resources /help-ing-hands/safe-sleep-practices-for-babies.

Nemours KidsHealth. Tummy time (for parents). Nemours KidsHealth. https://kidshealth.org/en/parents/tummy-time.html.

NHS. Feelings, relationships and pregnancy. NHS. https://www.nhs.uk /pregnancy/support/feelings-and-relationships/.

Pampers. How to implement an eat-play-sleep schedule for your baby. Pampers. https://www.pampers.com/en-us/baby/sleep/article/eat-play-sleep-schedule-for-baby.

Postpartum Depression Association. Paternal postpartum depression: PPD in men & how to cope. PostpartumDepression.org. https://www.postpartumdepression.org/postpartum-depression/men/.

Pregnancy Birth and Baby. Making a birth plan - what to include, purpose, benefits. Pregnancy Birth and Baby. https://www.pregnancybirthbaby.org.au/making-a-birth-plan.

Pregnancy Birth and Baby. Supporting your partner during her pregnancy. Pregnancy Birth and Baby. https://www.pregnancybirthbaby.org.au/supporting-your-partner-during-pregnancy.

Raising Children Network. Baby cues and baby body language: Video guide. Raising Children Network. https://raisingchildren.net.au/newborns/connecting-communicating/communicating/baby-cues.

Raising Children Network. Parenting teamwork: Why it's important. Raising Children Network. https://raisingchildren.net.au /grown-ups/looking-after-yourself/parenting/parenting-team-work#:~:text=For%20example%2C%20when%20parents%20see,impor-tant%20for%20children's%20emotional%20development.

The Bump. 8 ways to keep the spark alive in your relationship after baby. The Bump. https://www.thebump.com/a/revving-up-your-sex-life-after-baby.

TheBump.com. (2023, October 19). What Is a Birth Plan and Why Is It Important? https://www.thebump.com/a/tool-birth-plan#3.

The Gottman Institute. How we used the aftermath of a fight to repair our relationship. The Gottman Institute. https://www.gottman.com/blog/how-we-used-the-aftermath-of-a-fight-to-repair-our-relationship/.

UNICEF. Skin-to-skin contact - Baby Friendly Initiative. UNICEF. https://www.unicef.org.uk/babyfriendly/baby-friendly-resources/implementing-standards-resources/skin-to-skin-contact/.

Verywell Mind. Healthy communication tips - Relationships. Verywell Mind. https://www.verywellmind.com/managing-conflict-in-relationships-communication-tips-3144967.

WebMD Editors. 7 to 9 months pregnant - 3rd trimester baby growth. WebMD. https://www.webmd.com/baby/pregnancy-your-babys-growth-development-months-7-to-9.

What to Expect Editors. How to support your partner during pregnancy. What to Expect.https://www.whattoexpect.com/pregnancy/dads-guide/support-partner-during-pregnancy/.

Wirecutter. The best diapers. The New York Times. https://www.nytimes.com/wirecutter/reviews/best-diapers/.

Author Biography

Lane Carter is an energetic dad of three who brings his passion for sports and teamwork into the world of fatherhood. A former college athlete and lifelong sports enthusiast, Lane knows that being a great dad is a lot like being a great teammate and coach—it's all about preparation, strategy, and showing up when it counts.

With years of experience coaching youth sports and mentoring new dads, Lane is dedicated to helping first-time fathers train for the most important season of their lives: parenthood. His book breaks down the stages of pregnancy and early fatherhood into easy-to-follow game plans and checklists, helping Dad Rookies build confidence, mentally stay in the game, and support their partners like true MVPs.

Lane's mission is to make fatherhood approachable, exciting, and rewarding. He believes that, just like in sports, practice and patience lead to success—and that even the best dads fumble sometimes. His book provides play-by-play advice, pro tips and tricks, and encouragement to help new dads feel confident and game-day ready.

His passion for teamwork, commitment, and fatherhood shines through in his writing, making his guide a game-changing, go-to resource for dads looking to step up, stay strong, and enjoy every moment of fatherhood.